Advancing Student Knowledge in Cancer Epidemiology: New Insights and Perspectives

Ulrike Wagner

Copyright © [2023]

Title: Advancing Student Knowledge in Cancer Epidemiology: New Insights and Perspectives

Author's: Ulrike Wagner.

This book was printed and published by [Publisher's: Ulrike Wagner] in [2023]

ISBN:

TABLE OF CONTENTS

Chapter 1: Introduction to Cancer Epidemiology

Understanding Cancer Epidemiology

Cancer epidemiology is a branch of epidemiology that focuses on studying the patterns, causes, and effects of cancer in populations. It plays a crucial role in identifying risk factors, developing prevention strategies, and improving cancer control efforts. This subchapter aims to provide students with a comprehensive understanding of cancer epidemiology and its significance in the field of epidemiology.

The field of cancer epidemiology investigates the distribution and determinants of cancer in populations. It involves analyzing large sets of data to identify trends, patterns, and potential causes of cancer. By studying the occurrence of cancer in different populations, researchers can identify risk factors, such as age, gender, genetics, lifestyle choices, environmental exposures, and socio-economic factors.

Cancer epidemiology provides valuable insights into the burden of cancer on society. It helps researchers estimate the number of new cancer cases and deaths, assess the impact of cancer on different populations, and evaluate the effectiveness of cancer prevention and control measures. This information is essential for policymakers, healthcare professionals, and researchers to develop targeted interventions and allocate resources efficiently.

In this subchapter, students will learn about the various study designs used in cancer epidemiology, including cohort studies, case-control studies, and cross-sectional studies. They will gain knowledge about the strengths, limitations, and applications of each study design in investigating cancer-related questions.

Furthermore, students will be introduced to key concepts in cancer epidemiology, such as incidence, prevalence, mortality, survival rates, and cancer staging. They will understand how these measures are used to assess the burden, trends, and outcomes of cancer in populations.

Additionally, the subchapter will cover important topics in cancer epidemiology, such as cancer risk assessment, cancer screening, cancer surveillance, and cancer disparities. Students will explore the role of genetics, lifestyle factors, occupational and environmental exposures, and infectious agents in the development of cancer.

Finally, the subchapter will highlight the emerging trends and challenges in cancer epidemiology, including the impact of the aging population, advances in technology and data analysis, and the need for interdisciplinary collaborations.

Overall, this subchapter aims to equip students with a solid foundation in cancer epidemiology, enabling them to contribute to the field and make informed decisions in cancer prevention, control, and research. By understanding the patterns and determinants of cancer, students can play a vital role in reducing the burden of this devastating disease on individuals and communities.

Importance of Studying Cancer Epidemiology

Cancer has become a significant public health concern worldwide, and its impact on individuals and communities cannot be underestimated. As students venturing into the field of epidemiology, understanding the importance of studying cancer epidemiology is crucial. This subchapter aims to shed light on the significance of this field and its relevance to students interested in epidemiology.

Firstly, studying cancer epidemiology provides students with an opportunity to contribute to the prevention and control of cancer. By understanding the factors that contribute to the development and progression of cancer, students can identify preventive measures and interventions that can reduce the burden of the disease. Cancer epidemiology equips students with the necessary knowledge and skills to conduct research, analyze data, and implement evidence-based strategies to combat cancer.

Secondly, cancer epidemiology offers students a unique perspective on the multifaceted nature of cancer. This field explores how various factors, such as genetics, lifestyle choices, environmental exposures, and socioeconomic factors, interact to influence cancer development. By studying cancer epidemiology, students gain a comprehensive understanding of the complex interplay between biological, behavioral, and environmental factors in cancer causation.

Furthermore, cancer epidemiology provides students with an opportunity to make a significant impact on public health policy and practice. Through their research and analysis, students can generate valuable evidence that informs policymakers and healthcare professionals about the most effective strategies for cancer prevention and control. By studying cancer epidemiology, students become agents of change, driving evidence-based decision-making and improving cancer outcomes at the population level.

Additionally, studying cancer epidemiology opens doors to various career opportunities. As the field of cancer research continues to expand, there is a growing demand for skilled professionals in epidemiology. Students with expertise in cancer epidemiology can pursue careers in research institutions, government agencies, non-profit organizations, and academic settings. Moreover, they can contribute to global efforts in cancer control by working on international projects and collaborating with experts from diverse backgrounds.

In conclusion, the importance of studying cancer epidemiology cannot be overstated for students interested in the field of epidemiology. By understanding the factors contributing to cancer development, students can actively contribute to cancer prevention and control efforts. Moreover, studying cancer epidemiology provides students with a comprehensive understanding of the multifaceted nature of cancer and equips them with the skills to make a significant impact on public health policy and practice. With the growing demand for expertise in this field, students specializing in cancer epidemiology can pursue fulfilling careers and actively contribute to addressing the global burden of cancer.

Historical Overview of Cancer Epidemiology

Cancer is a complex disease that has plagued human populations for centuries. To understand the current state of cancer epidemiology, it is essential to delve into its historical roots and trace the evolution of our understanding of this disease. This subchapter aims to provide students with a comprehensive historical overview of cancer epidemiology, offering new insights and perspectives on the subject.

The history of cancer epidemiology can be traced back to ancient civilizations, where physicians observed cases of tumors and attempted to categorize them based on their physical characteristics. However, it was not until the late 19th century that the field of cancer epidemiology truly began to take shape. At that time, researchers started documenting the prevalence of cancer in different populations and started to recognize certain risk factors associated with the disease.

One of the most notable breakthroughs in cancer epidemiology occurred in the early 20th century when researchers discovered a link between tobacco smoking and lung cancer. This discovery revolutionized the field and paved the way for further investigations into the relationship between lifestyle factors and cancer risk. Subsequent studies identified additional risk factors such as exposure to environmental toxins, dietary patterns, and occupational hazards.

As the field of epidemiology advanced, so did our understanding of the various types of cancer. Researchers started to recognize that different cancers have distinct risk factors and patterns of occurrence. This realization led to the development of specialized subfields within cancer epidemiology, such as breast cancer epidemiology, colorectal cancer epidemiology, and so on.

In recent years, technological advancements have further propelled the field of cancer epidemiology forward. The advent of high-throughput sequencing technologies, for example, has allowed researchers to investigate the role of genetic factors in cancer development. Additionally, the use of large-scale population databases and data mining techniques has enabled researchers to uncover novel risk factors and patterns of cancer occurrence.

This subchapter aims to provide students with a comprehensive overview of the historical milestones in cancer epidemiology. By understanding the evolution of the field, students can gain a deeper appreciation for the current state of knowledge and the ongoing efforts to combat this devastating disease. Through new insights and perspectives, students can contribute to advancing our understanding of cancer epidemiology and ultimately make a difference in the prevention and treatment of cancer.

Key Concepts in Cancer Epidemiology

Cancer epidemiology is a branch of epidemiology that focuses on the study of cancer occurrence, patterns, and causes within populations. It plays a critical role in understanding the distribution and determinants of cancer, which in turn aids in the development of effective prevention and control strategies. This subchapter aims to introduce students to key concepts in cancer epidemiology, providing them with a foundation to further explore this field.

Incidence and Mortality Rates: One of the fundamental concepts in cancer epidemiology is the measurement of cancer occurrence. Incidence refers to the number of newly diagnosed cases of cancer within a population during a specific time period, usually expressed as the number of cases per 100,000 individuals. Mortality rate, on the other hand, represents the number of deaths caused by cancer within a population.

Risk Factors: Understanding the risk factors associated with cancer is crucial for prevention efforts. Risk factors may be classified into two main categories: modifiable and non-modifiable. Modifiable risk factors, such as tobacco use, diet, physical activity, and exposure to environmental carcinogens, can be altered through behavioral changes or public health interventions. Non-modifiable risk factors, such as age, gender, family history, and genetic predisposition, cannot be changed but can help identify individuals at higher risk.

Cancer Surveillance: Cancer surveillance is the ongoing, systematic collection, analysis, and interpretation of cancer data. It provides valuable information on cancer trends, patterns, and disparities, aiding in the identification of high-risk populations and informing public health policies. Students will learn about various surveillance systems, such as cancer registries, which collect data on cancer incidence, treatment, and outcomes.

Cancer   Screening:
Early detection of cancer through screening programs significantly improves treatment outcomes. This section will cover the principles and effectiveness of different cancer screening methods, including mammography for breast cancer, Pap tests for cervical cancer, and colonoscopy for colorectal cancer. Students will gain insights into the benefits and limitations of screening, as well as the importance of adherence to screening guidelines.

Cancer   Prevention   and   Control:
The ultimate goal of cancer epidemiology is to prevent and control cancer. This section will explore primary, secondary, and tertiary prevention strategies, including lifestyle modifications, vaccination programs (e.g., HPV vaccine), and targeted therapies. Students will learn about the role of epidemiology in evaluating the effectiveness of interventions and policies aimed at reducing cancer burden.

In summary, this subchapter on key concepts in cancer epidemiology provides students with a comprehensive introduction to the field. By covering incidence and mortality rates, risk factors, cancer surveillance, screening, and prevention and control strategies, students will gain a solid foundation for further exploration and research in this crucial area of epidemiology.

Chapter 2: Cancer Basics

Introduction to Cancer

Cancer is a complex and multifaceted disease that affects millions of people worldwide. It is a leading cause of death and is responsible for a significant burden on healthcare systems globally. Understanding the basics of cancer is crucial for students in the field of epidemiology, as it provides a foundation for studying the patterns, causes, and prevention of this devastating disease.

This subchapter aims to introduce students to the fundamental concepts of cancer, its prevalence, and the impact it has on individuals, communities, and society as a whole. By gaining a comprehensive understanding of cancer, students will be better equipped to contribute to the field of cancer epidemiology and develop innovative approaches to combat this disease.

The subchapter begins by defining cancer and explaining its characteristics. Cancer is a group of diseases characterized by the uncontrolled growth and spread of abnormal cells. It can occur in any part of the body and has the potential to invade nearby tissues and metastasize to distant organs. Students will learn about the different types of cancer, including carcinomas, sarcomas, lymphomas, and leukemias, and their respective origins within the body.

The chapter then explores the global burden of cancer, presenting statistics on its prevalence, incidence, and mortality rates. Students will gain insights into the impact of cancer on different populations, including variations in cancer rates based on age, gender, socioeconomic status, and geographical location. Understanding these factors is essential for identifying high-risk populations and implementing targeted prevention strategies.

Next, the subchapter delves into the major risk factors associated with cancer development. Students will learn about the role of genetics, environmental exposures, lifestyle choices, and infections in increasing cancer susceptibility. Emphasis is placed on the importance of modifiable risk factors, such as tobacco use, poor diet, physical inactivity, and alcohol consumption, which can be targeted through public health interventions.

Finally, the subchapter concludes by highlighting the significance of cancer epidemiology in improving cancer prevention and control. Students will be introduced to various study designs and methodologies used in epidemiological research to investigate the causes and risk factors of cancer. The role of cancer registries, surveillance systems, and data analysis in monitoring cancer trends and evaluating the effectiveness of interventions will also be discussed.

By the end of this subchapter, students will have a solid foundation in the field of cancer epidemiology, enabling them to pursue further studies and research in this important area. Armed with this knowledge, they will be well-equipped to contribute to the development of new insights and perspectives that can lead to better cancer prevention, early detection, and treatment strategies.

Cancer Development and Progression

Understanding the process of cancer development and progression is essential for students studying epidemiology. This subchapter aims to provide new insights and perspectives on the complex mechanisms involved in the formation and spread of cancer cells.

Cancer is a multifactorial disease that arises from a combination of genetic, environmental, and lifestyle factors. It begins with the transformation of normal cells into cancerous cells, a process known as carcinogenesis. This transformation is driven by genetic mutations that disrupt the normal control mechanisms of cell growth and division.

The subchapter starts by discussing the initiation stage of cancer development. It explores the various factors that can induce genetic mutations, including exposure to carcinogens such as tobacco smoke, radiation, and certain chemicals. Students will gain an understanding of how these mutations can lead to the activation of oncogenes, which promote uncontrolled cell proliferation, and the inactivation of tumor suppressor genes, which normally prevent the development of cancer.

Moving on to the progression stage, the subchapter delves into the mechanisms that enable cancer cells to invade neighboring tissues and metastasize to distant sites. Students will learn about the critical role of angiogenesis, the formation of new blood vessels, in providing nutrients and oxygen to growing tumors. The subchapter also explores the role of the immune system in recognizing and eliminating cancer cells, as well as the strategies employed by cancer cells to evade immune surveillance.

Furthermore, the subchapter highlights the importance of early detection and diagnosis in improving cancer outcomes. It introduces students to the concepts of tumor staging and grading, which help determine the extent of cancer spread and its aggressiveness. Students will also learn about the different diagnostic tools and screening methods available, such as imaging techniques and biomarker analysis.

To conclude, this subchapter provides students with a comprehensive overview of cancer development and progression, equipping them with the necessary knowledge to study and analyze the epidemiology of cancer. By understanding the underlying mechanisms, students will be better equipped to design and implement effective prevention and control strategies, ultimately contributing to the field of cancer epidemiology.

Types of Cancer

Cancer is a complex and diverse disease that affects millions of people worldwide. As students exploring the field of epidemiology, it is important to have a comprehensive understanding of the different types of cancer and their characteristics. This subchapter aims to provide you with a brief overview of some common types of cancer, highlighting their epidemiological aspects and shedding light on the challenges faced in studying them.

1. Breast Cancer: Breast cancer is the most prevalent cancer in women worldwide. Epidemiological studies have identified risk factors such as age, family history, hormonal factors, and lifestyle choices. Understanding the distribution of breast cancer and its risk factors is crucial in developing effective prevention and early detection strategies.

2. Lung Cancer: Lung cancer is one of the leading causes of cancer-related deaths globally. Tobacco smoking is the primary risk factor for lung cancer. Epidemiologists play a vital role in studying the impact of smoking cessation programs, occupational exposures, and environmental factors to reduce the burden of this disease.

3. Colorectal Cancer: Colorectal cancer affects the colon and rectum and is influenced by lifestyle factors, genetics, and age. Epidemiological research focuses on early detection methods, screening programs, and investigating the role of diet and physical activity in preventing this type of cancer.

4. Prostate Cancer: Prostate cancer primarily affects men, and the incidence increases with age. Epidemiological studies explore risk

factors, such as family history, race, and lifestyle choices. Identifying high-risk populations and developing targeted interventions are essential in reducing the impact of this disease.

5. Skin Cancer: Skin cancer, including melanoma and non-melanoma types, is strongly linked to exposure to ultraviolet (UV) radiation from the sun. Epidemiologists study the impact of preventive measures, such as sun protection programs and public awareness campaigns, to minimize the occurrence of skin cancer.

6. Leukemia: Leukemia is a cancer of the blood and bone marrow. Epidemiological research focuses on identifying potential environmental and genetic risk factors, as well as studying the impact of various treatment modalities on survival rates.

These are just a few examples of the numerous types of cancer that exist. Epidemiology plays a crucial role in understanding the distribution, risk factors, and prevention strategies for different cancers. By studying the epidemiology of cancer, students can contribute to the development of effective public health policies, early detection methods, and treatment interventions that can ultimately reduce the burden of cancer on individuals and societies. The challenges faced in studying cancer epidemiology, such as confounding factors, selection bias, and long-term follow-up, highlight the need for rigorous research methods and interdisciplinary collaboration in this field.

Common Risk Factors for Cancer

Cancer is a complex disease that affects millions of people worldwide. It is characterized by the uncontrolled growth and spread of abnormal cells in the body. While cancer can develop in any part of the body, certain risk factors increase the likelihood of its occurrence. Understanding these risk factors is crucial for students studying epidemiology, as it allows them to identify and analyze patterns of cancer occurrence within populations. In this subchapter, we will explore the common risk factors associated with cancer and their implications in the field of epidemiology.

1. Age: Advancing age is one of the most significant risk factors for cancer. As individuals grow older, the risk of developing cancer increases. This may be due to accumulated genetic mutations and exposure to environmental factors over time.

2. Tobacco Use: Smoking tobacco, including cigarettes, pipes, and cigars, is a leading cause of various types of cancer, such as lung, throat, mouth, and bladder cancer. Students need to be aware of the harmful effects of tobacco and its impact on cancer incidence.

3. Diet and Nutrition: Poor dietary choices, including a high intake of processed foods, red and processed meats, and low consumption of fruits and vegetables, have been linked to an increased risk of certain cancers, such as colorectal and stomach cancer. Understanding the role of nutrition in cancer development is essential for epidemiologists.

4. Physical Inactivity: Sedentary lifestyles contribute to the development of cancer. Lack of regular physical activity has been

associated with an increased risk of breast, colon, and endometrial cancer. Students should emphasize the importance of promoting an active lifestyle to reduce cancer risk.

5. Environmental Factors: Exposure to certain environmental hazards, such as air pollution, radiation, chemicals, and asbestos, can significantly increase the risk of cancer. Epidemiologists play a vital role in identifying and studying these environmental factors to develop preventive strategies.

6. Family History and Genetics: Some individuals may inherit gene mutations that make them more susceptible to certain types of cancer. Students should be familiar with the principles of genetic epidemiology and the identification of familial cancer syndromes.

7. Infectious Agents: Certain infections, such as human papillomavirus (HPV), hepatitis B and C viruses, and human immunodeficiency virus (HIV), have been linked to an increased risk of developing specific types of cancer. Understanding the role of infectious agents in cancer causation is critical for effective prevention and control strategies.

By understanding these common risk factors for cancer, students can contribute to the field of epidemiology by studying the distribution and determinants of cancer incidence. This knowledge enables the development of targeted interventions and policies aimed at reducing the burden of cancer within populations.

Chapter 3: Principles of Epidemiology

Introduction to Epidemiology

Epidemiology is a fascinating field that plays a crucial role in understanding the patterns and causes of diseases within populations. In this subchapter, we will delve into the world of epidemiology, providing students with a comprehensive introduction to this discipline and its significance in studying cancer.

Epidemiology can be defined as the study of the distribution and determinants of diseases in populations. It encompasses the investigation of various factors, including biological, environmental, and social determinants, to comprehend the occurrence and spread of diseases. By examining these factors, epidemiologists aim to identify risk factors, develop preventive measures, and ultimately improve public health outcomes.

The importance of epidemiology in the context of cancer research cannot be overstated. Cancer is a complex and multifaceted disease, and understanding its epidemiology is fundamental to developing effective prevention and control strategies. Epidemiologists employ various study designs, including cohort studies, case-control studies, and clinical trials, to gather data and analyze cancer trends. By examining the distribution of cancer cases across different populations, they are able to identify patterns and risk factors associated with specific types of cancer.

In this subchapter, we will begin by exploring the historical development of epidemiology, tracing its roots back to the work of pioneers such as John Graunt and John Snow. We will also discuss the fundamental concepts and principles that underpin epidemiological research, including measures of disease frequency, association, and causation. Understanding these concepts is essential for students to critically appraise and interpret epidemiological studies.

Next, we will delve into the various study designs and methodologies commonly employed in epidemiology. We will examine their strengths and limitations, providing students with the tools to choose the most appropriate design for specific research questions.

Furthermore, we will explore the role of epidemiology in cancer surveillance, screening, and prevention. Students will gain insights into the challenges faced in cancer epidemiology, such as biases, confounding, and the interpretation of statistical analyses.

By the end of this subchapter, students will have a solid understanding of the principles and methods of epidemiology and their application in cancer research. They will be equipped with the knowledge and skills necessary to critically evaluate epidemiological studies and contribute to the advancement of cancer epidemiology.

In conclusion, this subchapter serves as an introduction to the captivating world of epidemiology, with a specific focus on its relevance to cancer research. It provides students with a solid foundation to explore the intricacies of this field and encourages them to pursue further studies in epidemiology to advance our understanding of cancer and improve public health.

Study Designs in Cancer Epidemiology

Cancer epidemiology is a vital field of study that aims to understand the causes, distribution, and prevention of cancer in populations. To achieve this, researchers employ various study designs that provide valuable insights into the relationship between risk factors and the development of cancer. In this subchapter, we will explore the different study designs commonly used in cancer epidemiology.

1. Case-Control Studies: Case-control studies are retrospective in nature and involve comparing individuals with cancer (cases) to a control group without cancer. Researchers then look back at the past exposures and characteristics of both groups to identify potential risk factors. Case-control studies are particularly useful when studying rare cancers or diseases with long latency periods. However, they may be prone to recall bias and have limitations in establishing causality.

2. Cohort Studies: Cohort studies are prospective and involve following a group of individuals over time to assess their exposure to certain risk factors and cancer incidence. Researchers collect data on exposure and follow the cohort for an extended period to observe the development of cancer. Cohort studies allow for a more direct assessment of causality and can measure multiple outcomes. However, they can be time-consuming and expensive.

3. Cross-Sectional Studies: Cross-sectional studies are conducted at a specific point in time to determine the prevalence of cancer and its associated risk factors. Researchers collect data on a representative sample of the population and analyze the relationship between exposure and disease prevalence. Cross-sectional studies provide a

snapshot of the population, but they cannot establish temporal relationships or causality.

4. Ecological Studies: Ecological studies examine the relationship between cancer rates and population-level exposures. Researchers analyze data at the group or population level rather than individual level. Ecological studies utilize existing data sources, such as cancer registries and national databases, to assess the association between exposure and cancer incidence. While ecological studies can generate hypotheses, they cannot establish causal relationships at the individual level.

5. Clinical Trials: Clinical trials are experimental studies that evaluate the effectiveness of interventions or treatments in preventing or treating cancer. These studies involve randomly assigning participants to different treatment groups and comparing their outcomes. Clinical trials are essential for evidence-based medicine and contribute to developing new cancer therapies. However, they may have ethical considerations and take a long time to yield results.

By understanding these study designs, students of epidemiology can critically analyze cancer research and contribute to the field by designing and conducting their studies. Each study design has its strengths and limitations, and researchers must carefully select the appropriate design based on the research question and available resources.

In conclusion, study designs in cancer epidemiology play a crucial role in unraveling the complex relationships between risk factors and cancer development. Case-control studies, cohort studies, cross-sectional studies, ecological studies, and clinical trials each offer unique insights into the field. As students, it is important to grasp the nuances and implications of these study designs to contribute effectively to cancer epidemiology research and ultimately make a positive impact on cancer prevention and control efforts.

Data Collection Methods in Cancer Epidemiology

Cancer epidemiology is a specialized field of study that aims to understand the causes, distribution, and prevention of cancer within populations. To achieve this, researchers employ various data collection methods that help gather crucial information about cancer incidence, risk factors, and outcomes. This subchapter will delve into the different data collection methods commonly used in cancer epidemiology, providing students with a comprehensive understanding of how data is gathered and analyzed in this field.

One of the primary data collection methods in cancer epidemiology is the use of population-based cancer registries. These registries systematically collect data on cancer cases, including information on patient demographics, tumor characteristics, and treatment outcomes. By analyzing the data from these registries, researchers can identify trends and patterns in cancer occurrence, enabling them to develop effective prevention and control strategies.

Another important data collection method is the use of surveys and questionnaires. These tools are used to gather information directly from individuals about various risk factors, such as smoking habits, dietary patterns, and family history of cancer. Surveys can be conducted through face-to-face interviews, phone interviews, or online platforms, depending on the study's design and target population. By collecting data on individual behaviors and characteristics, researchers can identify potential risk factors and their associations with cancer development.

Furthermore, epidemiologists often rely on medical records and administrative databases to collect data on cancer-related outcomes, such as mortality rates and treatment utilization. These sources provide valuable information on disease progression, treatment efficacy, and overall patient outcomes. By analyzing these data, researchers can assess the effectiveness of different interventions and identify areas for improvement in cancer care.

In recent years, technological advancements have also contributed to data collection in cancer epidemiology. For instance, electronic health records and wearable devices can provide real-time data on patient health status, treatment adherence, and lifestyle behaviors. These innovative methods offer researchers a wealth of data, allowing them to examine the impact of various factors on cancer incidence and outcomes.

In conclusion, data collection methods play a vital role in cancer epidemiology, enabling researchers to identify risk factors, understand cancer patterns, and evaluate interventions. Population-based cancer registries, surveys, medical records, and emerging technologies all contribute to gathering comprehensive and accurate data. As students studying epidemiology, understanding these data collection methods will equip you with the necessary skills to contribute to the field and make a meaningful impact in cancer research and prevention efforts.

Measures of Association in Cancer Epidemiology

In the field of cancer epidemiology, understanding the measures of association is essential for identifying and quantifying the relationships between various risk factors and the occurrence of cancer. These measures provide valuable insights into the magnitude and direction of the associations, helping researchers and public health professionals make informed decisions and develop effective prevention strategies.

One commonly used measure of association in cancer epidemiology is the relative risk (RR). The relative risk compares the risk of developing cancer in individuals exposed to a specific risk factor to those who are not exposed. A relative risk greater than 1 indicates an increased risk, while a relative risk less than 1 suggests a decreased risk. This measure allows researchers to assess the strength of the association between a specific risk factor and cancer development.

Another measure of association is the odds ratio (OR), which is often used in case-control studies. The odds ratio compares the odds of exposure to a risk factor in cases (individuals with cancer) to the odds of exposure in controls (individuals without cancer). Similar to the relative risk, an odds ratio greater than 1 indicates an increased risk, while an odds ratio less than 1 suggests a decreased risk. The odds ratio is particularly useful when studying rare cancers or when the incidence rate is low.

Additionally, the attributable risk (AR) is a measure that quantifies the proportion of cancer cases in a population that can be attributed to a specific risk factor. It provides an estimate of the potential impact that eliminating or modifying a risk factor would have on reducing the burden of cancer. The attributable risk can be further divided into the population attributable risk (PAR), which considers the entire population, and the attributable fraction (AF), which focuses on the exposed population.

When interpreting measures of association, it is important to consider potential biases and confounding factors that may influence the results. Epidemiology students must be aware of the limitations and potential sources of error in order to accurately interpret and communicate the findings.

Understanding the measures of association in cancer epidemiology is crucial for students in the field of epidemiology as they contribute to the development of evidence-based cancer prevention and control strategies. By comprehending the magnitude and direction of associations between risk factors and cancer, students can identify high-risk populations, target interventions, and promote public health initiatives that aim to reduce the burden of cancer in communities.

Overall, measures of association provide vital information in cancer epidemiology. They allow researchers to quantify the relationships between risk factors and cancer occurrence, aiding in the identification of prevention strategies and the implementation of effective public health interventions. By grasping these measures, students in epidemiology can play a significant role in advancing our understanding of cancer etiology and ultimately contribute to reducing the global burden of cancer.

Chapter 4: Analyzing Cancer Data

Cancer Data Sources

Understanding cancer epidemiology requires access to reliable and comprehensive data sources. In this subchapter, we will explore the various types of data sources that students can utilize to advance their knowledge in cancer epidemiology.

1. Cancer Registries: Cancer registries are one of the primary sources of cancer data. These databases collect information on cancer cases, including patient demographics, tumor characteristics, treatment details, and outcomes. National and regional cancer registries play a crucial role in monitoring cancer trends and developing evidence-based strategies for cancer control. Students can access these registries to study cancer incidence, mortality rates, and survival rates in different populations.

2. Surveillance Systems: Public health surveillance systems provide valuable data on cancer-related risk factors, screening practices, and health behaviors. These systems collect information through surveys, questionnaires, and health records. By analyzing surveillance data, students can gain insights into the prevalence of risk factors such as smoking, obesity, and exposure to environmental carcinogens.

3. Cancer Research Databases: Numerous research databases house a wealth of information on cancer epidemiology. These databases contain data from clinical trials, cohort studies, case-control studies, and other research methodologies. Students can utilize these databases to analyze the associations between cancer risk factors, genetic factors,

and disease outcomes. Examples of cancer research databases include the Surveillance, Epidemiology, and End Results (SEER) program, the National Cancer Institute's (NCI) Cancer Genome Atlas (TCGA), and the International Agency for Research on Cancer (IARC) Data Portal.

4. Health Surveys: Population-based health surveys, such as the National Health Interview Survey (NHIS) and the Behavioral Risk Factor Surveillance System (BRFSS), provide data on a wide range of health conditions, including cancer. These surveys capture information on self-reported cancer diagnoses, cancer screening behaviors, and access to healthcare services. Students can analyze these survey data to explore disparities in cancer outcomes across different demographic groups and geographic regions.

5. Electronic Health Records (EHRs): With the widespread adoption of electronic health records, researchers now have access to vast amounts of clinical data. EHRs contain information on patient demographics, medical history, diagnostic tests, and treatment plans. Students can utilize EHR data to examine cancer treatment patterns, adherence to clinical guidelines, and the effectiveness of interventions.

By utilizing these various cancer data sources, students can gain a comprehensive understanding of cancer epidemiology. These sources provide a wealth of information on cancer incidence, mortality, risk factors, and treatment outcomes. With the knowledge gained from analyzing these data, students can contribute to the development of effective cancer prevention and control strategies, ultimately making a significant impact on public health.

Data Management and Quality Control

In the field of epidemiology, accurate and reliable data is crucial for conducting meaningful research and drawing valid conclusions. Data management and quality control play a vital role in ensuring the integrity of epidemiological studies. This subchapter aims to provide students with insights and perspectives on these essential aspects of data collection and analysis.

Data management involves various processes, including data collection, organization, storage, and retrieval. Students must understand the importance of using standardized data collection tools and techniques to ensure consistency and comparability across different studies. They should also familiarize themselves with data management software and databases commonly used in epidemiological research.

Quality control is an integral part of data management, focusing on the accuracy, completeness, and reliability of the collected data. Students need to be aware of potential sources of error, such as measurement bias, confounding factors, and missing data. They should learn how to implement quality control measures, including data cleaning, validation, and verification, to minimize errors and enhance the validity of their findings.

One key concept in data management and quality control is data integrity. Students should understand the importance of maintaining data integrity throughout the research process. This includes ensuring the confidentiality and security of data, adhering to ethical guidelines, and complying with relevant data protection regulations. Students should also be aware of the principles of data sharing and the benefits of open science in advancing epidemiological research.

Moreover, this subchapter will discuss the role of data management and quality control in different study designs, such as cohort studies, case-control studies, and cross-sectional studies. Students will learn how to address potential biases and confounding factors specific to each study design, as well as strategies for handling missing data.

Lastly, the subchapter will emphasize the importance of continuous monitoring and evaluation of data management and quality control processes. Students should be encouraged to reflect on their own research practices and identify areas for improvement. By adopting a systematic approach to data management and quality control, students can contribute to the advancement of cancer epidemiology and make meaningful contributions to the field.

In conclusion, data management and quality control are fundamental aspects of epidemiological research. This subchapter provides students with essential insights and perspectives on best practices in data collection, organization, and analysis. By mastering these skills, students will be well-equipped to conduct rigorous and impactful research in the field of cancer epidemiology.

Descriptive Analysis in Cancer Epidemiology

Descriptive analysis is an essential tool in cancer epidemiology that allows researchers to gain a comprehensive understanding of the distribution and characteristics of cancer cases within a population. By examining various demographic, clinical, and geographical factors, descriptive analysis helps to identify patterns and trends, which in turn can inform further research, prevention strategies, and healthcare interventions.

One of the key objectives of descriptive analysis in cancer epidemiology is to determine the burden of cancer in a specific population. This involves calculating cancer incidence rates, prevalence, and mortality rates, which provide crucial information about the magnitude of the disease. These rates can be stratified by age, sex, race, and other relevant variables to identify disparities and inequalities in cancer outcomes.

In addition to assessing the overall burden of cancer, descriptive analysis also aims to characterize the distribution of cancer cases by different factors. This includes examining the types and subtypes of cancer prevalent in a population, as well as the stage at which cancers are diagnosed. By understanding the distribution of cancer types, researchers can identify potential risk factors, genetic predispositions, and environmental exposures that may contribute to the development of specific cancers.

Geographical analysis is another important aspect of descriptive analysis in cancer epidemiology. By mapping the spatial distribution of cancer cases, researchers can identify clusters or hotspots of cancer incidence. This information can help to identify environmental factors, occupational exposures, or lifestyle patterns that may be contributing to the higher incidence rates in certain areas. Geographical analysis can also assist in resource allocation and planning for cancer prevention and control measures.

Descriptive analysis in cancer epidemiology is not limited to the examination of quantitative data. It also involves qualitative analysis, which helps to provide a deeper understanding of the experiences and perceptions of individuals living with cancer. Qualitative methods, such as interviews and focus groups, can shed light on the psychosocial, cultural, and economic factors that influence cancer outcomes and help to identify areas for targeted interventions.

Overall, descriptive analysis plays a critical role in cancer epidemiology by providing a comprehensive picture of the burden, distribution, and characteristics of cancer within a population. By understanding the patterns and trends revealed through descriptive analysis, students in the field of epidemiology can contribute to the development of effective prevention strategies, early detection programs, and interventions for improving cancer outcomes.

Analytical Techniques in Cancer Epidemiology

In the field of epidemiology, understanding the causes and patterns of cancer is of utmost importance. Analytical techniques play a crucial role in unraveling the complexities associated with cancer and aiding in the development of effective prevention and control strategies. This subchapter titled "Analytical Techniques in Cancer Epidemiology" aims to provide students with a comprehensive overview of the various analytical methods employed in this field.

One of the primary analytical techniques used in cancer epidemiology is the case-control study design. This design involves comparing individuals with a specific cancer diagnosis (cases) to individuals without the disease (controls) to identify potential risk factors. Students will learn about the strengths and limitations of case-control studies, as well as the statistical methods used to analyze the data, such as odds ratios and confidence intervals.

Another important analytical technique covered in this subchapter is cohort studies. These studies follow a group of individuals over time, collecting data on exposures and health outcomes. Students will gain an understanding of how cohort studies can be used to investigate the relationship between various risk factors and cancer incidence. They will also explore different types of cohort studies, including prospective and retrospective designs, and learn about the statistical techniques, such as relative risks, used to analyze cohort data.

Additionally, this subchapter will delve into advanced analytical techniques commonly used in cancer epidemiology. Students will be introduced to survival analysis, which examines the time from cancer diagnosis to death or other events of interest. They will also explore meta-analysis, a statistical method that combines data from multiple studies to obtain more robust estimates of risk. Students will learn how to interpret forest plots and assess heterogeneity within meta-analyses.

Furthermore, this subchapter will touch upon the emerging field of molecular epidemiology, which integrates molecular biology techniques with traditional epidemiological methods. Students will gain insights into how biomarkers, genetic profiling, and gene-environment interactions can enhance our understanding of cancer etiology and prognosis.

In conclusion, "Analytical Techniques in Cancer Epidemiology" provides students with a comprehensive overview of the various analytical methods employed in the field. By understanding these techniques, students will be better equipped to contribute to the advancement of cancer epidemiology, ultimately leading to improved prevention, early detection, and treatment of cancer.

Chapter 5: Cancer Surveillance and Registries

Cancer Surveillance Programs

In the field of epidemiology, cancer surveillance programs play a crucial role in monitoring and understanding the patterns and trends of cancer occurrence in populations. These programs are essential for detecting new cases, tracking changes in cancer incidence, and evaluating the impact of various interventions and policies aimed at reducing the burden of cancer.

Cancer surveillance programs collect, analyze, and disseminate data on cancer incidence, mortality, and survival rates. By systematically collecting information on cancer cases from hospitals, clinics, pathology laboratories, and other healthcare providers, these programs provide a comprehensive picture of the cancer burden within a population. They also help identify disparities in cancer occurrence among different demographic groups, such as age, sex, race/ethnicity, and socioeconomic status.

The data collected through cancer surveillance programs enable epidemiologists to identify high-risk populations, pinpoint geographical areas with increased cancer rates, and identify potential environmental or occupational risk factors associated with specific types of cancer. This information can guide public health interventions, such as targeted screening programs, cancer prevention campaigns, and policies to reduce exposure to known carcinogens.

Moreover, cancer surveillance programs contribute to the evaluation of cancer prevention and control efforts. By comparing cancer rates before and after the implementation of interventions, epidemiologists can assess the effectiveness of various strategies and make evidence-based recommendations for future interventions.

For students interested in cancer epidemiology, understanding the role and functioning of cancer surveillance programs is critical. These programs provide a rich source of data for research and analysis, offering valuable insights into the distribution and determinants of cancer. By studying the data collected by cancer surveillance programs, students can gain a comprehensive understanding of the burden of cancer, its risk factors, and the impact of prevention and control measures.

In this subchapter, we will delve into the intricacies of cancer surveillance programs, including their objectives, methodologies, and challenges. We will explore the different types of cancer data collected, discuss the importance of data quality and standardization, and highlight the role of technology in enhancing cancer surveillance efforts. By the end of this subchapter, students will have a solid foundation in cancer surveillance and be equipped with the knowledge and skills needed to contribute to cancer research and prevention initiatives.

Cancer Registries and their Role

In the field of epidemiology, cancer registries play a vital role in advancing our understanding of cancer and its impact on public health. These registries are comprehensive databases that systematically collect and store information about cancer cases and their characteristics, providing valuable insights into the distribution and patterns of cancer occurrence.

The primary purpose of cancer registries is to monitor the occurrence and trends of cancer within a defined population. By collecting data on newly diagnosed cancer cases, registries can identify changes in cancer rates over time and track the effectiveness of prevention and control efforts. This information is crucial for policymakers, healthcare professionals, and researchers to develop evidence-based strategies to reduce the burden of cancer.

Cancer registries collect a wide range of data, including patient demographics, tumor characteristics, treatment modalities, and outcomes. This wealth of information allows researchers to examine various aspects of cancer epidemiology, such as demographic and socioeconomic disparities in cancer incidence, survival rates, and the impact of different treatment approaches on patient outcomes.

Moreover, cancer registries facilitate the identification of high-risk populations and the evaluation of potential risk factors for specific types of cancer. By linking cancer data with other databases, such as environmental or occupational exposure records, researchers can explore the association between certain exposures and cancer development. These findings can inform preventive measures and help guide public health interventions.

In addition to their research function, cancer registries also play a crucial role in cancer surveillance. By providing accurate and timely data on cancer incidence and mortality, registries enable the early detection of trends, outbreaks, or unusual patterns of cancer occurrence. This information allows public health authorities to allocate resources efficiently, prioritize screening programs, and implement targeted interventions to reduce cancer burden within a population.

For students studying epidemiology, cancer registries offer a rich source of data for research and analysis. By utilizing registry data, students can gain hands-on experience in analyzing cancer trends, conducting risk factor assessments, and evaluating the impact of interventions. This practical application of epidemiological principles enhances students' understanding of the field and equips them with essential skills for a career in cancer epidemiology.

In conclusion, cancer registries are indispensable tools in cancer epidemiology. They provide a wealth of data on cancer occurrence, patterns, and outcomes, facilitating research, surveillance, and the development of evidence-based strategies for cancer prevention and control. For students interested in the field of epidemiology, cancer registries offer valuable resources to deepen their knowledge and contribute to the fight against cancer.

Cancer Data Collection and Analysis by Registries

In the field of epidemiology, the collection and analysis of cancer data play a crucial role in understanding the burden of this disease and developing effective strategies for prevention, detection, and treatment. Cancer registries serve as invaluable resources for researchers, clinicians, and policymakers, providing comprehensive data on cancer incidence, mortality, and survival rates.

This subchapter aims to provide students in the field of epidemiology with an overview of cancer data collection and analysis by registries, highlighting the significance of these resources and the methodologies employed in their operation.

Cancer registries are population-based databases that systematically collect, manage, and analyze information on all cancer cases occurring within a defined geographic area. These registries ensure the completeness, accuracy, and timeliness of cancer data, enabling epidemiologists to identify trends, patterns, and disparities in cancer occurrence and outcomes. They also serve as a foundation for research studies, clinical trials, and public health interventions.

The subchapter will delve into the key components of cancer registries, including the sources of data, such as hospitals, pathology laboratories, and death certificates. It will also discuss how data are collected, processed, and coded to ensure standardization and comparability across different registries. The role of trained cancer registrars in data collection, quality control, and analysis will be emphasized, highlighting the importance of their expertise in maintaining accurate and reliable cancer data.

Furthermore, the subchapter will explore the various uses of cancer registry data in epidemiological research. It will discuss how these data can be utilized to estimate cancer incidence rates, evaluate risk factors, track changes in cancer trends over time, and evaluate the effectiveness of cancer control strategies. The subchapter will also touch upon the ethical considerations associated with the use of registry data, such as patient confidentiality and informed consent.

Overall, this subchapter aims to provide students in the field of epidemiology with a comprehensive understanding of cancer data collection and analysis by registries. By familiarizing themselves with the intricacies of these resources, students will be better equipped to contribute to the field of cancer epidemiology, ultimately advancing our knowledge of this complex disease and improving public health outcomes.

Challenges and Future Directions in Cancer Surveillance

As students pursuing knowledge in epidemiology, it is crucial to understand the challenges and future directions in cancer surveillance. Cancer remains one of the leading causes of death worldwide, and effective surveillance systems are essential to monitor and control its impact on public health. In this subchapter, we will explore the various challenges faced in cancer surveillance and discuss potential future directions to enhance our understanding and response to this global health burden.

One of the main challenges in cancer surveillance is the heterogeneity of cancer types. Cancer is a complex disease with numerous subtypes, each with its own unique characteristics and risk factors. This heterogeneity poses challenges in standardizing data collection, classification, and reporting. To overcome this, future directions in cancer surveillance should focus on improving the accuracy and consistency of cancer diagnoses and classifications through advancements in molecular profiling and precision medicine.

Another challenge is the underreporting and incomplete data in cancer surveillance systems. This can occur due to various reasons, such as lack of awareness among healthcare providers, limited access to healthcare services, and inadequate reporting mechanisms. To address this challenge, efforts should be made to enhance education and awareness among healthcare professionals regarding cancer reporting requirements. Additionally, the use of electronic health records and data linkage systems can help improve the completeness and timeliness of cancer surveillance data.

Furthermore, the integration of new technologies and data sources can revolutionize cancer surveillance. The advancements in genomics, bioinformatics, and big data analytics provide opportunities to improve our understanding of cancer etiology, early detection, and treatment. Future directions in cancer surveillance should explore the use of these technologies to develop predictive models, identify high-risk populations, and tailor interventions based on individual risk profiles.

Additionally, addressing disparities in cancer surveillance is essential. Cancer incidence and mortality rates vary across different populations and socioeconomic groups. It is crucial to identify and understand these disparities to ensure equitable access to cancer prevention, early detection, and treatment services. Future directions in cancer surveillance should focus on collecting and analyzing data on social determinants of health, implementing targeted interventions, and promoting health equity in cancer care.

In conclusion, the challenges and future directions in cancer surveillance are multifaceted and require a multidisciplinary approach. As students in epidemiology, it is essential to recognize these challenges and contribute to the advancement of cancer surveillance by exploring new technologies, improving data collection and reporting systems, and addressing disparities in cancer care. By doing so, we can contribute to the global efforts in reducing the burden of cancer and improving the overall health outcomes for individuals and communities worldwide.

Chapter 6: Risk Factors and Prevention

Modifiable Risk Factors for Cancer

Cancer is a complex disease that affects millions of people worldwide. While some risk factors for cancer, such as age and family history, cannot be changed, there are several modifiable risk factors that students in the field of epidemiology should be aware of. By understanding these factors, students can play a crucial role in developing preventive strategies and interventions to reduce cancer incidence.

1. Tobacco Use: Smoking is the leading cause of preventable cancer deaths. Students should understand the harmful effects of smoking and the importance of promoting tobacco control measures such as public smoking bans, education campaigns, and support for smoking cessation programs.

2. Diet and Nutrition: Poor dietary choices, such as a high intake of processed foods, red meat, and sugary beverages, have been linked to an increased risk of several types of cancer. Students should explore the role of a healthy diet rich in fruits, vegetables, whole grains, and lean proteins in cancer prevention.

3. Physical Inactivity: Sedentary lifestyles contribute to the risk of developing certain cancers. Encouraging regular physical activity among individuals of all ages can help reduce the incidence of cancer. Students should explore the impact of exercise on cancer prevention and advocate for policies that promote active living.

4. Alcohol Consumption: Excessive alcohol consumption is a significant risk factor for various cancers, including breast, liver, and colorectal cancer. Students should be aware of the recommended limits for alcohol consumption and the potential benefits of alcohol reduction or abstinence.

5. Obesity: Obesity is associated with an increased risk of multiple cancers, including breast, colorectal, and pancreatic cancer. Students should examine the role of obesity in cancer development and explore strategies for promoting healthy weight management.

6. Environmental Factors: Exposure to certain environmental pollutants and occupational hazards can increase the risk of cancer. Students should investigate the impact of environmental factors, such as air pollution, chemicals, and radiation, on cancer incidence and advocate for policies that prioritize environmental health.

By understanding and addressing these modifiable risk factors, students can contribute to the development of effective public health campaigns, policies, and interventions to reduce the burden of cancer. Through their knowledge of epidemiology, students have the power to make a significant impact in preventing cancer and improving population health.

Non-Modifiable Risk Factors for Cancer

In the field of cancer epidemiology, it is crucial to understand the various risk factors that contribute to the development of this deadly disease. While some risk factors can be modified through lifestyle changes, there are certain factors that are beyond our control. These non-modifiable risk factors play a significant role in the occurrence of cancer and are essential knowledge for students studying epidemiology.

Genetics is one of the most prominent non-modifiable risk factors for cancer. Our genetic makeup determines our susceptibility to certain types of cancer. Inherited gene mutations can significantly increase the likelihood of developing specific cancers, such as breast, ovarian, colorectal, and prostate cancer. Understanding the role of genetics in cancer development is vital for students as it allows them to identify high-risk individuals and develop targeted prevention strategies.

Another non-modifiable risk factor for cancer is age. The risk of developing cancer increases with age, as our cells accumulate genetic mutations and become less efficient in repairing DNA damage. Students need to recognize the impact of aging on cancer incidence and understand the importance of early detection and screening in older populations.

Gender is also an important non-modifiable risk factor for certain cancers. For instance, breast cancer is predominantly seen in females, while prostate cancer is more common in males. Hormonal differences between genders contribute to these disparities, and students must grasp the nuances of gender-specific cancer risks to devise effective prevention and screening programs.

Race and ethnicity can also influence cancer risk. Certain racial and ethnic groups have a higher incidence of specific cancers due to a combination of genetic, environmental, and socioeconomic factors. For instance, African Americans have a higher risk of developing prostate and colorectal cancer compared to other ethnic groups. Recognizing these disparities is crucial for students to address health inequities and develop targeted interventions.

While non-modifiable risk factors cannot be changed, understanding their significance allows students in epidemiology to identify high-risk populations, implement effective screening programs, and develop strategies for early detection and prevention. By gaining insights into the role of genetics, age, gender, and race/ethnicity in cancer risk, students can contribute to reducing the burden of cancer on society.

In conclusion, this subchapter on non-modifiable risk factors for cancer provides students with a comprehensive understanding of the factors that contribute to cancer development beyond individual control. By expanding their knowledge on genetics, age, gender, and race/ethnicity, students can better design interventions and policies to tackle cancer at both individual and population levels.

Primary Prevention Strategies

In the field of epidemiology, primary prevention strategies play a crucial role in reducing the incidence of cancer and promoting overall health and well-being. These strategies focus on interventions that aim to prevent the initial development of cancer by targeting risk factors and promoting healthy behaviors. By implementing these strategies, students in the field of epidemiology can become powerful agents of change in reducing the burden of cancer in their communities and beyond.

One of the key primary prevention strategies is promoting healthy lifestyle choices. Research has consistently shown that certain behaviors, such as smoking, excessive alcohol consumption, poor diet, and lack of physical activity, significantly increase the risk of developing various types of cancer. Students in epidemiology can educate individuals and communities about the importance of adopting healthy behaviors, such as quitting smoking, eating a balanced diet rich in fruits and vegetables, engaging in regular physical activity, and moderating alcohol consumption. By raising awareness about these risk factors and promoting healthy choices, students can contribute to preventing cancer at its roots.

Another important primary prevention strategy is vaccination. Certain types of cancer, such as cervical and liver cancer, can be prevented through vaccination against human papillomavirus (HPV) and hepatitis B virus (HBV), respectively. Students in epidemiology can advocate for the importance of vaccination and work with healthcare providers and policymakers to ensure that vaccines are accessible and affordable for all individuals, especially in underserved communities.

Additionally, primary prevention strategies involve identifying and addressing environmental and occupational risk factors. Students in epidemiology can conduct research to identify potential carcinogens in the environment and workplaces, assess the associated risks, and work towards implementing regulations and policies to minimize exposure. By promoting clean air, safe drinking water, and occupational safety measures, students can contribute to reducing the incidence of cancer in the population.

In conclusion, primary prevention strategies are vital in the field of epidemiology for reducing the burden of cancer. By promoting healthy lifestyle choices, advocating for vaccination, and addressing environmental and occupational risk factors, students in epidemiology can make a significant impact on preventing cancer and improving overall health outcomes. Through their knowledge and dedication, they can contribute to creating a healthier future for individuals and communities around the world.

Secondary and Tertiary Prevention in Cancer Epidemiology

In the field of cancer epidemiology, prevention plays a crucial role in reducing the burden of this disease. While primary prevention focuses on preventing the occurrence of cancer altogether, secondary and tertiary prevention strategies aim to detect and treat cancer at its early stages and improve the quality of life for cancer survivors.

Secondary prevention in cancer epidemiology involves the early detection and diagnosis of cancer. This is typically done through screening programs that target individuals who are at a higher risk of developing certain types of cancer. For example, mammography is widely used for the early detection of breast cancer in women over the age of 40. Other common screening tests include colonoscopy for colorectal cancer and Pap smear for cervical cancer. By detecting cancer in its early stages, healthcare professionals can intervene and provide timely treatment, increasing the chances of survival and reducing the need for more aggressive and costly treatments.

Tertiary prevention, on the other hand, focuses on improving the quality of life for cancer survivors. This includes providing survivorship care plans, which outline the recommended follow-up care and support services for individuals who have completed their cancer treatment. These plans aim to address the long-term physical, psychosocial, and emotional needs of cancer survivors. Rehabilitation programs may also be offered to help survivors regain their physical strength and function after treatment, including physical therapy, occupational therapy, and counseling services.

Additionally, tertiary prevention involves ongoing surveillance and monitoring of cancer survivors for any signs of cancer recurrence or the development of secondary cancers. Regular follow-up appointments and imaging tests can help detect any potential issues early on, allowing for prompt intervention and improving the chances of successful treatment.

For students interested in epidemiology, understanding the importance of secondary and tertiary prevention in cancer epidemiology is essential. By studying and researching these strategies, students can contribute to the development of effective screening programs, survivorship care plans, and interventions that can ultimately reduce the burden of cancer on individuals and society as a whole.

In conclusion, secondary and tertiary prevention strategies are vital components of cancer epidemiology. By focusing on early detection and treatment, as well as the long-term care and support for cancer survivors, these prevention measures contribute to improving outcomes and quality of life for those affected by cancer. As students in the field of epidemiology, it is crucial to continue advancing our knowledge in these areas and work towards implementing evidence-based interventions to reduce the impact of cancer on individuals and communities.

Chapter 7: Cancer Screening and Early Detection

Importance of Cancer Screening

Cancer is a leading cause of death worldwide, and its incidence continues to rise. It is estimated that nearly one in three individuals will develop cancer at some point in their lives. However, the good news is that early detection and treatment of cancer can significantly improve survival rates. This is where cancer screening plays a vital role.

Cancer screening refers to the process of testing individuals who do not have any symptoms for the early detection of cancer. It aims to identify cancer at an early stage when it is most treatable, thus reducing the burden of the disease. Epidemiologists play a crucial role in understanding the impact of cancer screening on population health and developing effective screening programs.

There are several types of cancer screening tests available, including mammography for breast cancer, Pap test for cervical cancer, colonoscopy for colorectal cancer, and PSA test for prostate cancer, among others. These tests can detect cancer at its earliest stages or even detect pre-cancerous conditions, allowing for timely intervention and treatment. Regular cancer screening can help identify cancer before it spreads and increases the chances of successful treatment and survival.

Epidemiologists study the effectiveness of different cancer screening programs and evaluate their impact on reducing cancer-related morbidity and mortality. They analyze data from large population-based studies to determine the overall benefit of screening, including the potential harms such as false-positive results and overdiagnosis. By understanding the epidemiology of cancer and the impact of screening, students in the field of epidemiology can contribute to improving screening guidelines and policies.

Moreover, cancer screening is not only important for individuals but also for public health as a whole. Early detection and treatment of cancer can lead to a significant reduction in healthcare costs associated with advanced-stage cancer treatment. Additionally, effective screening programs can help identify high-risk populations and implement targeted interventions to reduce cancer disparities.

In conclusion, cancer screening is of utmost importance in the field of epidemiology. It plays a critical role in identifying cancer at its earliest stages, enabling timely treatment and improving survival rates. By studying the impact of screening programs, epidemiologists can contribute to the development of effective guidelines and policies that can reduce the burden of cancer on both individuals and society. As students in the field of epidemiology, it is essential to understand the significance of cancer screening and actively contribute to advancing knowledge in this area to improve cancer outcomes.

Types of Cancer Screening Tests

Cancer screening tests play a crucial role in the early detection and prevention of various types of cancer. As students in the field of epidemiology, it is essential to have a comprehensive understanding of the different screening tests available to identify and diagnose cancer in its early stages. This subchapter will discuss the various types of cancer screening tests and their significance in cancer epidemiology.

1. Mammography: Mammograms are X-ray examinations used to detect breast cancer in women. This screening test is recommended for women aged 40 and above, as it can detect breast tumors even before they are palpable. Regular mammograms can significantly improve the chances of early detection, increasing the likelihood of successful treatment.

2. Pap Smear: Pap smears are used to detect cervical cancer in women. During this procedure, a small sample of cells is collected from the cervix to identify any abnormal changes. Regular Pap smears can identify pre-cancerous cells, allowing for prompt intervention and preventing the development of invasive cervical cancer.

3. Colonoscopy: Colonoscopy is a procedure that examines the large intestine and rectum for any abnormalities or signs of colorectal cancer. This screening test is crucial for individuals aged 45 and above, as it can detect precancerous polyps and remove them before they turn cancerous. Early detection through colonoscopies has proven to be effective in reducing mortality rates associated with colorectal cancer.

4. Prostate-Specific Antigen (PSA) Test: The PSA test is used to screen for prostate cancer in men. It measures the levels of PSA, a protein

produced by the prostate gland, in the blood. Elevated PSA levels may indicate the presence of prostate cancer or other prostate conditions. However, it is important to note that the PSA test may have limitations, and further diagnostic tests, such as biopsies, are often required for confirmation.

5. Lung Cancer Screening: Low-dose computed tomography (CT) scans are recommended for individuals at high risk of developing lung cancer, such as heavy smokers or those with a history of smoking. These scans can detect lung cancer in its early stages when it is more treatable.

It is vital for students in the field of epidemiology to understand the importance of cancer screening tests in identifying cancer early, as it allows for timely intervention and improved patient outcomes. However, it is crucial to note that cancer screening tests have limitations, including false positives and false negatives, and should always be accompanied by further diagnostic tests when necessary.

By familiarizing ourselves with the various types of cancer screening tests, we can contribute to the development of effective cancer prevention strategies and improve public health outcomes in cancer epidemiology.

Screening Programs and Guidelines

Screening programs and guidelines play a crucial role in the field of epidemiology, as they aim to detect cancer at an early stage, when it is more treatable and the chances of survival are higher. These programs are designed to identify individuals who may be at a higher risk of developing cancer or who already have early signs of the disease. By implementing effective screening programs, epidemiologists can help reduce the burden of cancer and improve overall population health.

One of the most widely recognized screening programs is for breast cancer, which primarily affects women. Guidelines recommend regular mammograms for women above a certain age, usually starting at 40 or 50 years old, depending on the country and specific risk factors. Mammograms are X-ray images of the breast that can identify tumors or other abnormalities. Through early detection, breast cancer screening programs have significantly contributed to decreasing mortality rates and improving treatment outcomes.

Similarly, cervical cancer screening programs have been successful in reducing the incidence and mortality of this type of cancer. Regular Pap smears or human papillomavirus (HPV) testing are recommended for women to identify any precancerous or cancerous changes in the cervix. HPV vaccination has also become an essential component of cervical cancer prevention programs, targeting young individuals before they become sexually active.

Colorectal cancer screening programs focus on detecting precancerous polyps or early-stage cancers in the colon or rectum. Guidelines typically recommend starting regular screenings with a colonoscopy or fecal occult blood test at the age of 50, although this may vary based on individual risk factors. These programs have demonstrated significant reductions in colorectal cancer mortality by identifying and removing precancerous polyps before they develop into cancer.

It is important for students in the field of epidemiology to understand the purpose, benefits, and limitations of various cancer screening programs. They should be familiar with the guidelines established by national and international organizations and be able to critically evaluate the evidence supporting different screening methods. Additionally, students should be aware of the challenges associated with implementing and promoting screening programs, such as accessibility, cost-effectiveness, and ethical considerations.

By gaining a comprehensive understanding of screening programs and guidelines, students of epidemiology can contribute to the development and improvement of effective cancer prevention strategies. With their knowledge and expertise, they can help shape policies and interventions that will ultimately reduce the burden of cancer and improve the health outcomes of populations worldwide.

Challenges in Cancer Screening Implementation

One of the primary goals of cancer epidemiology is to identify effective strategies for early detection and prevention. Cancer screening plays a crucial role in achieving this objective, as it aims to identify the disease at an early stage when treatment is more effective. However, the implementation of cancer screening programs is not without its challenges. In this subchapter, we will explore some of the common obstacles faced in the implementation of cancer screening and the importance of addressing them.

One significant challenge in cancer screening implementation is the lack of awareness and knowledge among the general population. Many individuals may not fully understand the importance of screening or may have misconceptions about the procedure. Educating the public about the benefits and risks of cancer screening is crucial to increasing participation rates and ensuring its success. Students studying epidemiology have a unique opportunity to contribute to this effort by spreading accurate information and debunking myths surrounding cancer screening.

Another challenge is the accessibility and affordability of screening services. In many regions, particularly low-income areas, access to screening facilities may be limited, leading to disparities in cancer detection and outcomes. Students can play a vital role in advocating for improved access to screening services, especially in underserved communities. They can also explore innovative approaches, such as mobile screening units or telemedicine, to reach individuals who face barriers to traditional screening settings.

Furthermore, the effectiveness of cancer screening programs relies heavily on the quality and accuracy of screening tests. False-positive and false-negative results can have significant consequences, including unnecessary invasive procedures or delayed diagnosis. Students studying epidemiology can contribute to improving the reliability of screening tests by conducting research on new screening technologies or evaluating the performance of existing methods.

Additionally, the ethical considerations surrounding cancer screening implementation should not be overlooked. Balancing the benefits and potential harms of screening, ensuring informed consent, and protecting individual privacy are critical aspects that need to be addressed. Students can engage in discussions and research on ethical issues related to cancer screening, contributing to the development of guidelines and policies that prioritize patient well-being.

In conclusion, while cancer screening is a vital tool in cancer epidemiology, its successful implementation is not without challenges. Lack of awareness, limited access, quality concerns, and ethical considerations are all hurdles that need to be overcome. As students studying epidemiology, it is essential to recognize these challenges and actively work towards addressing them to improve the effectiveness and equity of cancer screening programs. By doing so, we can make significant strides in early detection and prevention, ultimately reducing the burden of cancer on individuals and communities.

Chapter 8: Cancer Treatment and Survival

Cancer Treatment Modalities

Cancer treatment has come a long way over the years, with various modalities being developed to target and combat this deadly disease. In this subchapter, we will explore the different treatment options available for cancer patients, providing students with an in-depth understanding of the various modalities used in cancer epidemiology.

One of the most common treatment modalities is surgery, which involves removing the tumor from the body. Surgery can be curative, especially when cancer is detected at an early stage and has not spread to other parts of the body. It can also be used in combination with other treatments such as chemotherapy or radiation therapy to ensure the best possible outcome for the patient.

Chemotherapy is another widely used cancer treatment modality. It involves the administration of drugs to kill or slow down the growth of cancer cells. These drugs can be given orally or intravenously, and they target rapidly dividing cells, which include cancer cells. Chemotherapy is often used in cases where surgery is not an option or to destroy any remaining cancer cells after surgery.

Radiation therapy is another important modality in cancer treatment. It uses high-energy radiation to kill cancer cells or shrink tumors. This treatment is usually delivered externally through a machine called a linear accelerator, which targets the affected area precisely, minimizing damage to healthy tissues surrounding the tumor. Radiation therapy can be used alone or in combination with other treatment modalities, depending on the type and stage of cancer.

Immunotherapy is a relatively new and promising cancer treatment modality that aims to boost the body's immune system to fight cancer cells. It involves the use of drugs that stimulate the immune system or genetically modify immune cells to recognize and attack cancer cells. Immunotherapy has shown great potential in treating various types of cancers and has revolutionized cancer treatment in recent years.

Targeted therapy is another modality that focuses on specific characteristics of cancer cells, such as genetic mutations or proteins unique to cancer cells. By targeting these specific characteristics, targeted therapy aims to inhibit the growth and spread of cancer cells, with minimal impact on healthy cells.

In conclusion, understanding the different treatment modalities available for cancer patients is crucial in the field of cancer epidemiology. Surgery, chemotherapy, radiation therapy, immunotherapy, and targeted therapy are all important tools in the fight against cancer. As students, it is essential to comprehend the strengths, limitations, and potential side effects of each modality to contribute to the advancement of cancer treatment and improve patient outcomes.

Cancer Treatment Outcomes and Survival Rates

Understanding the outcomes of cancer treatment and the survival rates associated with different types of cancer is crucial in the field of epidemiology. As students studying cancer epidemiology, it is essential to gain insights into the current landscape of cancer treatment and the factors that influence patient outcomes.

Cancer treatment outcomes refer to the effectiveness of various treatment modalities in managing and curing cancer. These outcomes are often measured by survival rates, which indicate the percentage of patients who survive for a specific period after diagnosis or treatment. Survival rates provide valuable information on the success of different treatment approaches and help researchers identify areas for improvement.

It is important to note that survival rates can vary significantly depending on the type and stage of cancer, as well as individual patient characteristics. Factors such as age, overall health, and access to healthcare services can also impact survival outcomes. Epidemiologists play a vital role in analyzing these factors to understand the disparities in cancer treatment outcomes among different populations.

In recent years, advancements in cancer research and treatment have led to improved survival rates for many types of cancer. Early detection, personalized medicine, and targeted therapies have revolutionized cancer treatment, resulting in higher survival rates for specific cancers, such as breast, prostate, and colorectal cancer.

However, challenges still exist in achieving optimal outcomes for all cancer patients. Some types of cancer, such as pancreatic and lung cancer, remain particularly challenging to treat, with lower survival rates compared to other malignancies. Identifying the reasons behind these disparities and developing innovative strategies to improve outcomes for these cancer types is a critical area of research within cancer epidemiology.

Moreover, studying long-term survivorship and the impact of treatment on survivors' quality of life is another important aspect of cancer epidemiology. Understanding the potential long-term effects of cancer treatment can help healthcare providers and policymakers develop comprehensive survivorship care plans and support systems for cancer survivors.

In conclusion, cancer treatment outcomes and survival rates are fundamental aspects of cancer epidemiology. As students in this field, gaining a comprehensive understanding of the factors that influence these outcomes and the disparities that exist among different populations is essential. With continued research and advancements in cancer treatment, the goal of improving survival rates and ensuring optimal outcomes for all cancer patients can be achieved.

Factors Affecting Cancer Treatment Success

Cancer treatment success is influenced by a variety of factors that researchers and healthcare professionals in the field of epidemiology have been studying for decades. Understanding these factors is crucial for students pursuing a career in cancer epidemiology as it provides valuable insights into the challenges faced by patients and the healthcare system in achieving positive treatment outcomes. This subchapter explores some of the key factors that affect the success of cancer treatments, shedding light on the complexities of this field.

One of the primary factors affecting cancer treatment success is early detection. The earlier cancer is diagnosed, the higher the chances of successful treatment. Screening programs and public awareness campaigns play a vital role in ensuring early detection, allowing for prompt intervention and improved survival rates. Students studying epidemiology should be aware of the importance of early detection in the fight against cancer.

Another crucial factor is access to quality healthcare services. Disparities in healthcare access and utilization have been shown to significantly impact cancer treatment outcomes. Socioeconomic factors, geographical location, and health insurance coverage all play a role in determining the availability and affordability of cancer treatments. Students should understand these disparities and work towards addressing them to ensure equitable access to cancer care.

Furthermore, the effectiveness of cancer treatments can be influenced by individual patient characteristics. Factors such as age, gender, genetic predisposition, and overall health status can impact treatment response and overall prognosis. Epidemiologists study these factors to identify population subgroups that may require tailored treatment approaches to improve outcomes.

In addition to individual factors, the type and stage of cancer also play a vital role in treatment success. Different cancers respond differently to various treatment modalities, and the stage at which cancer is diagnosed affects treatment options and success rates. Students should familiarize themselves with the various cancer types and their specific treatment considerations to contribute to the development of personalized and effective treatment approaches.

Lastly, ongoing research and advancements in cancer treatment technologies are constantly shaping the landscape of cancer care. Students should stay updated with the latest breakthroughs in cancer treatment, including targeted therapies, immunotherapies, and precision medicine approaches. Keeping abreast of these advancements will enable students to contribute to the development and implementation of innovative treatment strategies.

In conclusion, understanding the factors that affect cancer treatment success is crucial for students in the field of cancer epidemiology. Early detection, access to quality healthcare, individual patient characteristics, cancer type and stage, and advancements in treatment technologies all impact treatment outcomes. By studying these factors and working towards addressing disparities, students can contribute to improving cancer treatment success rates and ultimately reducing the burden of cancer on individuals and communities.

Survivorship and Quality of Life in Cancer Epidemiology

Cancer epidemiology is a field of study that focuses on understanding the distribution, causes, and prevention of cancer in populations. It plays a crucial role in informing public health policies and interventions to reduce the burden of cancer. However, the impact of cancer extends beyond its incidence and mortality rates. Survivorship and quality of life are important aspects that need to be addressed in cancer epidemiology, particularly as more individuals are living longer after a cancer diagnosis.

Survivorship refers to the period after cancer treatment ends, encompassing the physical, emotional, and social issues faced by cancer survivors. With advancements in early detection and treatment, the number of cancer survivors has been increasing steadily. This presents unique challenges and opportunities for epidemiologists to explore the long-term effects of cancer and its treatments. By studying survivorship, researchers can identify risk factors that may influence the development of late effects, such as secondary cancers or chronic health conditions.

Quality of life is another crucial dimension to consider in cancer epidemiology. It encompasses various aspects, including physical functioning, psychological well-being, social relationships, and overall satisfaction with life. Cancer and its treatments can have a significant impact on a person's quality of life, affecting their ability to perform daily activities, work, and engage in social activities. Understanding the factors that influence quality of life can help inform interventions to improve the well-being of cancer survivors.

Epidemiologists studying survivorship and quality of life in cancer epidemiology employ a range of research methods, including population-based surveys, longitudinal studies, and qualitative research. These approaches allow for a comprehensive assessment of the physical, psychological, and social factors that influence survivorship outcomes and quality of life.

In this subchapter, we will delve into the various dimensions of survivorship and quality of life in cancer epidemiology. We will explore the challenges faced by cancer survivors, such as managing long-term side effects and psychological distress. Additionally, we will investigate the role of lifestyle factors, social support, and access to healthcare in influencing survivorship outcomes and quality of life.

By understanding the survivorship experiences and quality of life of cancer survivors, epidemiologists can contribute to the development of supportive care programs and interventions that address the unique needs of this population. This subchapter aims to offer insights and perspectives for students interested in advancing their knowledge in cancer epidemiology, particularly in the areas of survivorship and quality of life research.

Chapter 9: Emerging Trends and Innovations in Cancer Epidemiology

Molecular Epidemiology in Cancer Research

In recent years, there has been a significant shift in cancer research towards understanding the molecular basis of this complex disease. This emerging field, known as molecular epidemiology, combines traditional epidemiological methods with molecular biology techniques to unravel the intricate mechanisms behind cancer development and progression. As students of epidemiology, it is crucial to gain knowledge and insights into the fascinating world of molecular epidemiology in cancer research.

At its core, molecular epidemiology seeks to identify the genetic and environmental factors that contribute to the development of cancer. By studying the molecular alterations in tumors, researchers can uncover specific biomarkers, genetic mutations, and epigenetic modifications that can help predict an individual's risk of developing cancer and guide personalized treatment strategies.

One of the key advantages of molecular epidemiology is its ability to provide a deeper understanding of the heterogeneity of cancer. Through the analysis of various molecular markers, researchers can classify tumors into distinct subtypes, each with unique characteristics and treatment responses. This knowledge not only aids in the identification of high-risk individuals but also facilitates the development of targeted therapies that can improve patient outcomes.

Moreover, molecular epidemiology plays a crucial role in identifying potential environmental carcinogens. By studying the interactions between specific genetic variants and environmental exposures, researchers can identify individuals who are more susceptible to certain carcinogens. This information can then be used to implement preventive measures and reduce the burden of cancer in populations.

As students, it is essential to familiarize ourselves with the tools and techniques used in molecular epidemiology. From next-generation sequencing to gene expression profiling, understanding these methodologies will enable us to interpret and critically evaluate the latest research findings. Additionally, gaining knowledge in bioinformatics and data analysis will be invaluable in conducting robust molecular epidemiological studies.

In conclusion, molecular epidemiology in cancer research represents a paradigm shift in our understanding of this complex disease. By combining epidemiological methods with molecular biology techniques, researchers can unravel the underlying mechanisms of cancer development, identify high-risk individuals, and develop targeted therapies. As students of epidemiology, it is crucial to embrace this exciting field and equip ourselves with the necessary knowledge and skills to contribute to the ongoing advancements in molecular epidemiology.

Precision Medicine and Personalized Cancer Care

Advancements in technology and our understanding of the human genome have paved the way for a new era in cancer treatment and care. Precision medicine, a groundbreaking approach that tailors medical interventions to the individual characteristics of each patient, has revolutionized the field of oncology. In this subchapter, we will explore the concept of precision medicine and its application in personalized cancer care, particularly focusing on its relevance to students in the field of epidemiology.

Precision medicine is based on the understanding that each patient's genetic makeup, lifestyle, and environmental factors play a crucial role in determining their risk of developing cancer and their response to treatment. By analyzing a patient's unique genetic profile, healthcare professionals can identify specific genetic alterations that drive the growth and progression of cancer. This knowledge allows for the development of targeted therapies that selectively attack the cancer cells while sparing healthy tissues, minimizing side effects, and increasing treatment efficacy.

For students in the field of epidemiology, understanding precision medicine is essential as it provides valuable insights into the mechanisms underlying cancer development and progression. By studying the genetic alterations associated with specific cancer types, epidemiologists can identify high-risk populations and develop strategies for prevention and early detection. Furthermore, precision medicine offers the potential for more accurate prognostication and prediction of treatment response, enabling epidemiologists to design studies that evaluate the effectiveness of personalized treatments and interventions.

Personalized cancer care goes beyond genetic profiling and targeted therapies. It encompasses a multidisciplinary approach that takes into account each patient's unique circumstances, including their medical history, lifestyle, and preferences. This holistic approach recognizes that cancer is not a one-size-fits-all disease and emphasizes the importance of individualized care plans that consider the whole person.

In conclusion, precision medicine and personalized cancer care represent a paradigm shift in oncology, offering new avenues for prevention, treatment, and patient care. For students in the field of epidemiology, understanding the principles and applications of precision medicine is crucial for advancing our knowledge of cancer etiology, improving patient outcomes, and shaping future research and practice. By embracing this transformative approach, we can continue to make significant strides in the fight against cancer and ultimately improve the lives of patients worldwide.

Big Data and Artificial Intelligence in Cancer Epidemiology

In recent years, the field of cancer epidemiology has witnessed a revolutionary transformation with the advent of big data and artificial intelligence (AI). These innovative technologies have brought new insights and perspectives, enabling researchers and students to delve deeper into the understanding of cancer causation, prevention, and treatment. This subchapter explores the intersection of big data and AI in cancer epidemiology, highlighting their potential applications and impact on the field.

Big data refers to the vast amount of information generated from various sources, including electronic health records, genomics, social media, and wearable devices. This wealth of data provides a unique opportunity for cancer epidemiologists to uncover patterns, trends, and associations that were previously unattainable. By analyzing large datasets, researchers can identify risk factors, biomarkers, and genetic variations that contribute to cancer development and progression.

Artificial intelligence, on the other hand, encompasses a range of technologies such as machine learning, natural language processing, and computer vision. These AI tools can analyze complex datasets, recognize patterns, and make predictions, enabling researchers to develop personalized approaches to cancer prevention and treatment. For instance, machine learning algorithms can predict cancer risk based on a combination of genetic, environmental, and lifestyle factors, facilitating targeted interventions and early detection strategies.

One of the major applications of big data and AI in cancer epidemiology is precision medicine. By integrating genetic and clinical data, researchers can identify subgroups of patients who are more likely to respond to specific treatments, minimizing adverse effects and improving overall outcomes. Moreover, AI-powered predictive models can aid in the identification of high-risk populations, enabling healthcare providers to implement preventive measures and interventions at an early stage.

Another area where big data and AI have made significant contributions is in cancer surveillance and monitoring. By analyzing real-time data from various sources, including social media and wearable devices, researchers can track cancer trends, identify hotspots, and monitor the effectiveness of public health interventions. This real-time monitoring can facilitate the timely implementation of targeted cancer control measures, ultimately reducing the burden of the disease.

In conclusion, the integration of big data and artificial intelligence in cancer epidemiology has opened up new horizons for research and innovation. These technologies have the potential to revolutionize cancer prevention, diagnosis, and treatment by providing personalized and precise approaches. As students in the field of epidemiology, it is essential to embrace and harness the power of big data and AI to advance our knowledge and contribute to the fight against cancer. By leveraging these tools, we can uncover hidden patterns, develop targeted interventions, and ultimately make a significant impact on cancer control and patient outcomes.

Future Directions and Opportunities in Cancer Epidemiology

As students delve into the field of epidemiology, it is essential to understand the evolving landscape of cancer epidemiology. With advancements in technology, the discovery of new risk factors, and an increased understanding of molecular mechanisms, the future of cancer epidemiology holds immense potential for exciting discoveries and impactful interventions.

One of the key future directions in cancer epidemiology is the integration of big data and advanced analytics. The availability of large-scale datasets, such as electronic health records, genomics, and environmental data, presents an opportunity to uncover novel associations and patterns in cancer development. Students can explore the use of machine learning algorithms and artificial intelligence to identify high-risk populations, predict cancer outcomes, and develop personalized prevention strategies.

Another promising area of research is the exploration of the exposome, which encompasses the totality of environmental exposures throughout an individual's life. By comprehensively assessing the impact of various environmental factors, such as air pollution, occupational hazards, and lifestyle choices, on cancer risk, students can contribute to a more comprehensive understanding of the disease and inform preventive measures.

Furthermore, the advent of precision medicine and the increasing availability of molecular data provide a unique opportunity to advance cancer epidemiology. By integrating genetic and molecular information with epidemiological data, students can identify subtypes of cancer, understand their etiology, and develop targeted interventions. This approach has the potential to revolutionize cancer prevention, screening, and treatment strategies, leading to improved outcomes for patients.

In addition to these scientific advancements, there are several opportunities for students in the field of cancer epidemiology. Collaboration and interdisciplinary research are key to addressing the complex challenges associated with cancer. By working with experts from diverse fields, such as genetics, oncology, statistics, and public health, students can gain a broader perspective and contribute to innovative solutions.

Moreover, students can explore the role of social determinants of health in cancer disparities. Understanding how factors such as socioeconomic status, race, and access to healthcare contribute to differential cancer outcomes can help develop targeted interventions to reduce these disparities.

As students embark on their journey in cancer epidemiology, they should embrace the future directions and opportunities in the field. By harnessing the power of big data, advanced analytics, precision medicine, and interdisciplinary collaborations, they can make significant contributions to our understanding of cancer etiology, prevention, and control. With their passion and dedication, the next generation of epidemiologists holds the potential to make a profound impact on the global burden of cancer.

Chapter 10: Ethical Considerations in Cancer Epidemiology

Privacy and Confidentiality in Cancer Research

In the field of cancer research, privacy and confidentiality play a crucial role in ensuring the ethical conduct of studies and the protection of participants' rights. Epidemiology students embarking on a journey to contribute to this important field must understand the significance of maintaining privacy and confidentiality throughout their research endeavors.

Privacy refers to the individual's right to control the collection, use, and disclosure of their personal information. In cancer research, it is essential to respect this right by safeguarding participants' identities and any identifiable information they provide. Confidentiality, on the other hand, refers to the obligation of researchers to protect the data collected from participants and prevent unauthorized access or disclosure.

Respecting privacy and maintaining confidentiality are not only ethical imperatives but also legal requirements. Researchers must adhere to various regulations, such as the Health Insurance Portability and Accountability Act (HIPAA) in the United States, which ensures the privacy and security of individuals' health information. Students studying epidemiology must familiarize themselves with these regulations and ensure compliance throughout their research projects.

To safeguard privacy and maintain confidentiality, students should adopt several best practices. Firstly, obtaining informed consent from participants is essential. Informed consent ensures that participants understand the purpose of the study, the potential risks and benefits, and what will happen to their data. Students should explain how their data will be anonymized or de-identified to protect privacy.

Secondly, students should utilize secure data storage and transmission methods. This includes password-protected databases, encrypted communication channels, and restricted access to physical or electronic files. Regularly updating security measures and protocols is crucial to prevent data breaches.

Furthermore, researchers must be cautious when presenting or publishing research findings. They should avoid including any identifying information or use pseudonyms to further protect participants' privacy. Additionally, students should be aware of the potential risks of re-identification when sharing or linking datasets, especially in the era of big data and advanced computational methods.

Lastly, maintaining privacy and confidentiality also involves proper disposal of data. Once the research is complete, students should ensure that all data containing identifiable information is permanently deleted or securely destroyed.

In conclusion, privacy and confidentiality are paramount in cancer research, and students pursuing epidemiology must be well-versed in the ethical and legal considerations associated with these principles. By obtaining informed consent, utilizing secure data storage, practicing responsible data sharing, and appropriately disposing of data, students can contribute to cancer research while upholding the privacy rights of participants.

Informed Consent and Research Ethics

In the field of epidemiology, conducting research studies is crucial for advancing our understanding of diseases and developing effective strategies for prevention and treatment. However, it is essential to ensure that research is conducted ethically and with the informed consent of participants. This subchapter will explore the importance of informed consent and research ethics in cancer epidemiology.

Informed consent is the process by which individuals are provided with comprehensive information about a research study before deciding whether to participate. It is a fundamental ethical principle that respects individuals' autonomy and ensures their rights and welfare are protected. In cancer epidemiology, obtaining informed consent is particularly critical due to the sensitive nature of the research and potential risks involved.

When conducting research on cancer, epidemiologists must carefully explain to potential participants the purpose of the study, any potential risks or benefits, the confidentiality of the data collected, and their right to withdraw from the study at any time without repercussions. It is crucial that students in epidemiology understand the significance of obtaining informed consent and the ethical responsibility they hold as researchers.

Moreover, research ethics in cancer epidemiology extend beyond obtaining informed consent. Students must also consider the privacy and confidentiality of participants' data. Respecting participants' privacy is essential for maintaining their trust and ensuring that their personal information is not misused or disclosed without their consent. Students should be aware of the legal and ethical guidelines for handling and storing sensitive data, such as de-identifying information and securing data storage systems.

Furthermore, research ethics also involve ensuring the scientific integrity of the study. This means conducting research with honesty, accuracy, and transparency. Epidemiology students must adhere to rigorous research methods, accurately report their findings, and avoid any conflicts of interest that could compromise the validity of their research.

By understanding the principles of informed consent and research ethics, students in epidemiology can contribute to the field responsibly and ethically. This subchapter aims to equip students with the knowledge and skills necessary to conduct research studies that prioritize the rights, welfare, and informed decision-making of participants.

In conclusion, informed consent and research ethics play a vital role in cancer epidemiology. Students must understand the importance of obtaining informed consent, respecting privacy and confidentiality, and upholding scientific integrity. By adhering to these ethical principles, students can contribute to the advancement of knowledge in cancer epidemiology while ensuring the protection and well-being of research participants.

Ethical Challenges and Dilemmas in Cancer Epidemiology

Introduction:
In the field of cancer epidemiology, researchers encounter various ethical challenges and dilemmas that require careful consideration and decision-making. These challenges arise due to the sensitive nature of studying cancer in human populations and the potential impact of research findings on individuals and communities. This subchapter aims to provide insights into the ethical considerations that students in the field of epidemiology must be aware of and navigate when conducting cancer research.

Informed   Consent:
One of the fundamental ethical principles in cancer epidemiology is obtaining informed consent from study participants. Students must understand the importance of ensuring that individuals fully comprehend the purpose, risks, and benefits of participating in research studies. Informed consent should be obtained in an understandable language and tailored to the cultural and educational backgrounds of participants.

Confidentiality   and   Privacy:
Protecting the confidentiality and privacy of participants is crucial in cancer epidemiology. Students must be aware of the potential risks associated with collecting and storing sensitive health information. They should implement strict data protection measures, such as de-identification and encryption, to safeguard participants' identities and maintain confidentiality.

Equity   and   Justice:
Cancer epidemiology research should prioritize equity and justice in participant recruitment and study design. Students should consider the potential biases that may arise from disparities in access to healthcare, education, and socioeconomic status. They should strive to include diverse populations to ensure the generalizability of research findings and address health disparities.

Publication   and   Dissemination:
Ensuring responsible publication and dissemination of research findings is another ethical challenge in cancer epidemiology. Students must adhere to ethical guidelines and practices when reporting their results, including transparently disclosing conflicts of interest and avoiding exaggerated claims. Responsible dissemination of research findings can contribute to evidence-based decision-making and avoid potential harm caused by misinformation.

Community   Engagement:
Engaging with the community is crucial in cancer epidemiology research. Students should establish partnerships with community organizations and stakeholders to ensure that research is conducted in a culturally sensitive and respectful manner. Involving the community in the research process can enhance participant recruitment, improve study relevance, and facilitate knowledge translation.

Conclusion:
Ethical challenges and dilemmas are inherent in cancer epidemiology research. Students in the field of epidemiology must be aware of these challenges and strive to navigate them ethically. By upholding principles such as informed consent, confidentiality, equity,

responsible publication, and community engagement, students can contribute to the advancement of cancer epidemiology knowledge while respecting the rights and well-being of study participants.

87

Ethical Guidelines for Conducting Cancer Epidemiology Studies

Introduction:
Cancer epidemiology plays a crucial role in understanding the causes, distribution, and prevention of cancer in populations. As students in the field of epidemiology, it is essential to adhere to a set of ethical guidelines when conducting cancer epidemiology studies. These guidelines ensure the protection of human subjects, maintain the integrity of research, and promote responsible and transparent scientific practices.

Informed   Consent:
Obtaining informed consent is a fundamental ethical principle in research involving human subjects. Students should prioritize informed consent, ensuring that participants understand the purpose, risks, and benefits of the study. Communication should be clear, concise, and culturally sensitive, allowing participants to make an informed decision about their involvement while respecting their autonomy.

Confidentiality   and   Privacy:
Respecting the privacy and confidentiality of study participants is of utmost importance. Students must ensure that collected data are de-identified and stored securely, preventing unauthorized access or disclosure. Researchers should handle personal information responsibly, protecting the privacy rights of participants and maintaining confidentiality throughout the study and publication process.

Avoiding   Harm:
Students must strive to minimize any potential harm that may arise from their research. This includes carefully considering the potential physical, psychological, social, or economic risks associated with the study. Adequate measures should be taken to protect vulnerable populations, including children, pregnant women, or individuals with cognitive impairments, ensuring their well-being and minimizing any potential harm.

Scientific   Integrity:
Maintaining scientific integrity is vital in cancer epidemiology studies. Students should adhere to rigorous research methodologies, accurately collect and analyze data, and report findings truthfully and objectively. Any conflicts of interest should be disclosed, and research should be conducted with transparency, avoiding bias, and ensuring reproducibility.

Responsible   Data   Sharing:
Data sharing is an essential aspect of cancer epidemiology research. Students should consider making their data accessible to the scientific community, allowing for independent verification and replication of results. However, data sharing should be done responsibly, ensuring the protection of participant privacy and confidentiality.

Ethics   Review:
Students should seek approval from an ethics review board or institutional review board (IRB) before initiating their research. This ensures that the study design, methodology, and informed consent process meet ethical standards. Students should engage in ongoing

ethical review, seeking guidance from mentors or professional organizations when facing ethical dilemmas during their research.

Conclusion:

As students in the field of epidemiology, it is paramount to conduct cancer epidemiology studies with the highest ethical standards. Ethical guidelines ensure the protection of participants, maintain scientific integrity, and promote responsible and transparent research practices. By adhering to these guidelines, students contribute to the advancement of knowledge in cancer epidemiology and help improve public health outcomes.

Chapter 11: Translating Epidemiological Findings into Public Health Practice

Role of Epidemiology in Public Health

Epidemiology plays a crucial role in public health, serving as the foundation for understanding disease patterns, identifying risk factors, and implementing effective prevention and control strategies. In the field of cancer epidemiology, this discipline is particularly significant, as it helps researchers and public health officials gain insights into the causes and distribution of cancer in populations. This subchapter aims to provide students with an overview of the role of epidemiology in public health, emphasizing its importance in cancer research and prevention.

Epidemiology involves the study of disease occurrence and distribution in populations, as well as the identification of factors contributing to disease development. By analyzing data on cancer incidence, prevalence, and mortality rates, epidemiologists can identify trends and patterns that can guide public health interventions. They investigate the influence of various risk factors, such as genetic predisposition, lifestyle choices, environmental exposures, and socioeconomic factors on cancer development.

In the context of cancer epidemiology, students will learn about the different study designs employed to investigate the etiology of cancer, including cohort, case-control, and cross-sectional studies. They will understand the strengths and limitations of each design and how to interpret the results obtained.

Furthermore, students will explore the various analytical methods used in cancer epidemiology, such as calculating relative risks, odds ratios, and attributable risks. These statistical tools help quantify the association between exposures and cancer outcomes, allowing researchers to estimate the impact of specific risk factors on disease occurrence.

In addition to examining cancer etiology, students will also delve into the role of epidemiology in cancer prevention and control. They will learn about the importance of cancer screening programs, early detection strategies, and vaccination campaigns in reducing the burden of cancer. Epidemiologists also play a vital role in identifying disparities in cancer outcomes among different populations and developing targeted interventions to address these inequities.

Overall, this subchapter highlights the indispensable role of epidemiology in public health, specifically in the field of cancer epidemiology. By understanding the principles and methods of epidemiology, students can contribute to the advancement of cancer research, prevention, and control efforts, ultimately making significant contributions to improving global health outcomes.

Translational Research in Cancer Epidemiology

In the field of epidemiology, the study of cancer holds immense importance due to its impact on global health. Cancer epidemiology aims to understand the distribution, causes, and prevention strategies for cancer at a population level. Within this field, translational research plays a crucial role in bridging the gap between scientific discoveries and practical applications in cancer prevention and control.

Translational research refers to the process of translating scientific findings into real-world interventions and policies. It involves the application of knowledge gained from basic research and clinical trials to improve public health outcomes. In the context of cancer epidemiology, translational research focuses on translating epidemiological findings into effective cancer prevention and control strategies.

This subchapter explores the significance of translational research in cancer epidemiology and its impact on advancing our understanding of cancer etiology, prevention, and treatment. It delves into the various stages of translational research, from bench to bedside, and highlights the challenges and opportunities associated with each stage.

One of the key aspects of translational research in cancer epidemiology is the integration of multidisciplinary approaches. It involves collaboration between epidemiologists, clinicians, biostatisticians, and policymakers to ensure the effective translation of research findings. By bringing together experts from various fields, translational research in cancer epidemiology can tackle complex challenges and develop innovative solutions.

The subchapter also discusses the role of epidemiological studies in identifying risk factors for cancer and the subsequent translation of these findings into prevention strategies. It highlights the importance of rigorous study design, data collection, and analysis in generating reliable evidence for cancer prevention.

Furthermore, the subchapter explores the impact of translational research on cancer treatment. It discusses the use of epidemiological data to inform personalized medicine approaches, identify biomarkers for early detection, and assess the effectiveness of new therapies.

Overall, this subchapter provides a comprehensive overview of translational research in cancer epidemiology, emphasizing its role in advancing our knowledge of cancer etiology, prevention, and treatment. It aims to equip students in the field of epidemiology with a deeper understanding of the translational research process and its implications for improving cancer outcomes. By engaging with this subchapter, students will gain insights into the interdisciplinary nature of cancer epidemiology and the potential for innovative solutions in cancer prevention and control.

Policy Development and Implementation

Policy development and implementation play a crucial role in the field of epidemiology, as they provide a framework for addressing and managing public health issues, including cancer epidemiology. In this subchapter, we will explore the importance of policy development and implementation, and how it impacts students studying epidemiology.

Policy development involves the creation of guidelines, regulations, and procedures that aim to address specific public health concerns. In the context of cancer epidemiology, policies can be developed to promote cancer prevention, early detection, and treatment. These policies are essential in reducing the burden of cancer and improving the overall health outcomes of individuals affected by this disease.

For students studying epidemiology, understanding policy development is vital, as it provides a foundation for creating evidence-based strategies to combat cancer. By examining existing policies and their implementation, students can gain insights into the challenges and opportunities in public health decision-making. Moreover, they can learn about the role of various stakeholders, such as government agencies, non-profit organizations, and healthcare providers, in shaping and implementing these policies.

Implementation of policies is equally important, as it translates the theoretical framework into practical actions. Students need to be aware of the challenges associated with policy implementation, such as resource constraints, political considerations, and stakeholder engagement. By understanding the complexities of policy implementation, students can develop realistic and effective strategies to overcome these barriers.

Furthermore, this subchapter will highlight successful examples of policy development and implementation in cancer epidemiology. Case studies from different countries and regions will be discussed to provide students with a global perspective on how policies can impact cancer prevention and control. These examples will showcase the importance of interdisciplinary collaboration, community engagement, and advocacy in achieving successful policy outcomes.

To enhance the learning experience, this subchapter will also include interactive exercises and discussions. Students will be encouraged to critically analyze existing policies, propose improvements, and develop implementation plans. By actively engaging in these activities, students can develop the necessary skills and knowledge to contribute to policy development and implementation in their future epidemiological work.

In conclusion, policy development and implementation are fundamental aspects of epidemiology, particularly in the field of cancer epidemiology. This subchapter aims to equip students with the necessary knowledge and skills to understand, analyze, and contribute to policy development and implementation processes. By exploring real-life examples, discussing challenges, and engaging in interactive exercises, students will be better prepared to address public health issues and advance knowledge in cancer epidemiology.

Communicating Epidemiological Findings to the Public

As students delving into the field of epidemiology, it is crucial to understand the significance of effectively communicating epidemiological findings to the public. While research and data analysis are essential components of the epidemiological process, the ultimate goal is to improve public health outcomes by disseminating pertinent information to the broader population. This subchapter aims to equip students with the knowledge and skills necessary to communicate epidemiological findings in an accessible and impactful manner.

Epidemiological findings often hold critical insights into the causes, risk factors, and prevention strategies related to various diseases, including cancer. Communicating these findings effectively can empower individuals to make informed decisions regarding their health and well-being. However, translating complex scientific information into easily understandable language can be challenging. Therefore, it is essential to employ various communication strategies to bridge the gap between epidemiological research and the public.

One key aspect of communicating epidemiological findings is tailoring the message to the target audience. As students, it is imperative to recognize the diversity within the general public and adapt communication methods accordingly. Whether addressing healthcare professionals, policymakers, or the general public, selecting the appropriate language, tone, and medium can significantly impact the effectiveness of the communication.

Furthermore, visual aids such as infographics, charts, and graphs can enhance comprehension and engagement. Students should familiarize themselves with data visualization techniques and software to effectively present epidemiological findings. Visual representations not only simplify complex information but also make it more memorable and accessible to a wider audience.

Additionally, utilizing various communication channels is crucial in reaching different segments of the population. Social media platforms, websites, traditional media outlets, and community events are all valuable avenues for disseminating epidemiological findings. By embracing diverse communication channels, students can ensure that their research reaches and resonates with a wide range of individuals.

Lastly, maintaining transparency and acknowledging the limitations of epidemiological research is vital when communicating findings to the public. Clearly stating the uncertainties, potential biases, and evolving nature of scientific knowledge fosters trust and prevents misinformation or misconceptions from spreading.

In conclusion, effective communication of epidemiological findings is an essential skill for students in the field of epidemiology. By tailoring messages, utilizing visual aids, employing diverse communication channels, and maintaining transparency, students can bridge the gap between complex research and public understanding. Ultimately, the ability to effectively communicate epidemiological findings will contribute to improved public health outcomes and empower individuals to make informed decisions regarding their well-being.

Chapter 12: Future Directions in Cancer Epidemiology

Advancements in Technology and Cancer Epidemiology

In recent years, advancements in technology have revolutionized the field of cancer epidemiology, offering new insights and perspectives for students interested in this niche of epidemiology. From sophisticated data collection methods to innovative analytical tools, these technological advancements have significantly enhanced our understanding of cancer causes, risk factors, and prevention strategies.

One of the most significant advancements is the development of advanced data collection techniques. Traditionally, cancer epidemiologists relied on surveys and self-reported data, which often introduced biases and inaccuracies. However, with the advent of electronic health records (EHRs) and big data analytics, researchers now have access to vast amounts of real-time patient information. This enables them to conduct large-scale studies and track cancer trends more accurately, leading to more reliable and evidence-based conclusions.

Furthermore, the integration of genomic technology has had a profound impact on cancer epidemiology. The ability to sequence and analyze an individual's DNA has allowed researchers to identify specific genetic mutations associated with different types of cancer. This knowledge not only aids in understanding the underlying causes of cancer but also helps in developing personalized treatment plans and targeted prevention strategies.

Another remarkable advancement is the application of artificial intelligence (AI) and machine learning algorithms in cancer epidemiology. These technologies can analyze complex datasets, identify patterns, and predict cancer outcomes with high accuracy. AI can also assist in early detection and diagnosis by analyzing medical images and identifying potential cancerous lesions that may be missed by human observers. This integration of technology and epidemiology opens up new possibilities for improved cancer management and patient outcomes.

Moreover, mobile health applications and wearable devices have empowered individuals to actively participate in cancer prevention and management. These technologies allow real-time monitoring of lifestyle factors, such as physical activity, diet, and sleep patterns, which are known to influence cancer risk. With this information, individuals can make informed decisions about their health and take proactive measures to reduce their cancer risk.

In conclusion, the advancements in technology have revolutionized cancer epidemiology, providing students in this field with new insights and perspectives. From advanced data collection methods to genomic technology, artificial intelligence, and mobile health applications, these technological advancements have significantly enhanced our understanding of cancer causes and prevention strategies. As students in epidemiology, embracing these advancements and staying updated with emerging technologies will be essential to contribute to the ongoing fight against cancer.

Collaborative Research and International Cooperation

In the field of epidemiology, collaboration and international cooperation play a vital role in advancing knowledge and understanding of cancer. Research conducted in collaboration with experts from different countries and diverse backgrounds brings together a wealth of knowledge, expertise, and resources that can lead to groundbreaking discoveries and new perspectives in cancer epidemiology.

Collaborative research allows students in the field of epidemiology to expand their knowledge and gain exposure to different research methodologies, study designs, and data analysis techniques. By working together with researchers from around the world, students can enhance their understanding of the global burden of cancer and the various factors that contribute to its occurrence and progression. Additionally, collaborative research provides students with valuable opportunities to network and build professional relationships with experts in the field, which can open doors to future collaborations and career advancement.

International cooperation in cancer epidemiology is crucial for several reasons. Firstly, cancer is a global health issue that affects populations across different countries and regions. By fostering international cooperation, researchers can share data, resources, and best practices to develop a comprehensive understanding of cancer patterns and risk factors. This knowledge can then be used to inform public health policies and interventions on a global scale, leading to more effective cancer prevention and control strategies.

Moreover, international cooperation allows for the pooling of resources and expertise, enabling large-scale research projects that would be unfeasible for individual researchers or institutions. Through initiatives such as multinational cohort studies or collaborative meta-analyses, researchers can amass substantial amounts of data, leading to more robust and generalizable findings.

For students in epidemiology, international cooperation provides unique opportunities to engage in research projects on a global scale. By participating in international collaborations, students can contribute to cutting-edge research, gain exposure to diverse populations, and develop cross-cultural competencies that are increasingly valued in the field. Furthermore, international collaborations often offer access to funding opportunities, scholarships, and exchange programs, enabling students to broaden their horizons and enhance their professional development.

In conclusion, collaborative research and international cooperation are essential for advancing knowledge in cancer epidemiology. By working together across borders and disciplines, researchers in the field can make significant strides in understanding the causes, prevention, and control of cancer. For students in epidemiology, engaging in collaborative and international research not only expands their knowledge but also provides them with unique opportunities for personal and professional growth.

Interdisciplinary Approaches to Cancer Epidemiology

Cancer is a complex disease that affects millions of people around the world, making it one of the leading causes of death. Epidemiology, the study of how diseases spread and affect populations, plays a crucial role in understanding and combating cancer. However, in order to truly make progress in this field, it is essential to adopt interdisciplinary approaches.

Interdisciplinary approaches to cancer epidemiology involve integrating knowledge and methods from various disciplines, such as biology, genetics, statistics, and social sciences. This allows researchers to gain a more comprehensive understanding of the disease and its impact on different populations. By combining insights from different fields, students of epidemiology can expand their knowledge and develop new perspectives on cancer.

One important aspect of interdisciplinary approaches to cancer epidemiology is the integration of biological and genetic factors. Understanding the biological mechanisms underlying cancer development and progression is crucial for identifying risk factors and developing targeted prevention and treatment strategies. By combining genetic data with epidemiological studies, researchers can identify genetic variations that increase the risk of cancer, as well as gene-environment interactions that contribute to disease development.

Furthermore, incorporating statistical methods into cancer epidemiology allows for more robust analyses and interpretation of data. Students with a background in statistics can contribute significantly to the field by developing models and techniques to analyze large datasets, identify trends, and assess the effectiveness of interventions. Statistical methods also enable researchers to account for confounding factors and biases, ensuring more accurate results.

Another interdisciplinary approach to cancer epidemiology involves incorporating social sciences. Factors such as socioeconomic status, cultural beliefs, and access to healthcare play a significant role in cancer risk and outcomes. Studying the social determinants of health can provide valuable insights into health disparities and inform targeted interventions to reduce cancer burden in vulnerable populations.

In conclusion, interdisciplinary approaches to cancer epidemiology are essential for advancing our understanding of this complex disease. By integrating knowledge and methods from various disciplines, students of epidemiology can gain new insights and perspectives on cancer. Incorporating biology, genetics, statistics, and social sciences into cancer epidemiology allows for a more comprehensive analysis of the disease and its impact on different populations. By adopting interdisciplinary approaches, we can make significant progress in preventing, diagnosing, and treating cancer, ultimately improving the health outcomes of individuals and communities worldwide.

Promoting Student Engagement and Career Opportunities in Cancer Epidemiology

Cancer epidemiology is a fascinating and rapidly growing field that offers students a unique opportunity to make a significant impact on public health. This subchapter aims to highlight the importance of promoting student engagement in cancer epidemiology while shedding light on the various career opportunities available within this niche field.

Engaging students in cancer epidemiology is crucial as it not only fosters their interest and passion for public health but also equips them with the necessary skills and knowledge to tackle the challenges of cancer prevention and control. By actively involving students in research projects, internships, and hands-on experiences, educational institutions can cultivate a new generation of epidemiologists dedicated to reducing the burden of cancer worldwide.

One effective way of promoting student engagement is through mentorship programs. Establishing strong mentor-mentee relationships allows students to receive guidance from experienced professionals in the field. These mentors can provide valuable insights, share their experiences, and help students navigate the complexities of cancer epidemiology. Additionally, mentorship programs often offer networking opportunities, which can be instrumental in securing internships and future job placements.

Another avenue for student engagement is participation in conferences, workshops, and seminars focused on cancer epidemiology. These events provide students with the chance to learn from experts, present their own research findings, and engage in meaningful discussions with peers and professionals. Active involvement in such activities not only enhances their knowledge but also cultivates critical thinking and analytical skills essential for a successful career in cancer epidemiology.

Furthermore, internships and research assistantships in cancer epidemiology offer students practical experience and exposure to real-world challenges. These opportunities allow students to apply their theoretical knowledge, work alongside seasoned professionals, and contribute to ongoing research projects. Such experiences not only deepen their understanding of the field but also provide valuable networking connections and potential job prospects.

In terms of career opportunities, the field of cancer epidemiology offers a wide array of options. Graduates can pursue careers in academia, where they can conduct research, teach, and mentor future epidemiologists. Additionally, opportunities exist within government agencies, non-profit organizations, and private research institutions, where professionals play a vital role in policy development, program implementation, and data analysis to inform cancer prevention strategies.

In conclusion, promoting student engagement in cancer epidemiology is crucial for cultivating a passionate and skilled workforce dedicated to reducing the burden of cancer. By providing mentorship, offering opportunities for practical experience, and showcasing the diverse career paths available, educational institutions can inspire students to pursue a fulfilling career in this niche field. With their knowledge and expertise, future epidemiologists can make significant contributions to cancer prevention and control, ultimately improving public health outcomes for communities worldwide.

As students pursuing knowledge in the field of epidemiology, you have embarked on a journey that holds immense potential for making a difference in the global fight against cancer. In this subchapter, we will explore the captivating world of cancer epidemiology and delve into the various opportunities that await you in this exciting field.

Cancer epidemiology is a specialized branch of epidemiology that focuses on understanding the causes, patterns, and prevention of cancer in populations. It involves studying the distribution and determinants of cancer incidence, prevalence, and mortality, with the ultimate goal of informing public health strategies and interventions.

One of the key aspects of promoting student engagement in cancer epidemiology is fostering a deep understanding of its significance. By comprehending the impact of cancer on individuals, families, and societies, students can develop a strong motivation to contribute to cancer prevention and control efforts. This subchapter will provide you with compelling insights into the burden of cancer and the potential for making a difference through epidemiological research.

Additionally, we will explore the diverse career opportunities that exist in cancer epidemiology. From academic research to public health agencies, pharmaceutical companies, and non-profit organizations, the field offers a wide range of rewarding paths. You will discover how your skills in data analysis, research design, and critical thinking can be applied to tackle pressing issues in cancer prevention and control, such as identifying risk factors, evaluating screening and treatment strategies, and monitoring population-level trends.

Furthermore, this subchapter will highlight the importance of networking and collaboration in advancing your career in cancer epidemiology. By nurturing connections with experienced professionals and engaging in interdisciplinary collaborations, you can gain valuable insights, access resources, and enhance your research capabilities.

To support your journey in cancer epidemiology, we will also provide recommendations for further education and training opportunities. Whether it is through advanced degree programs, workshops, or online courses, continuous learning and skill development are essential to stay at the forefront of this rapidly evolving field.

In conclusion, this subchapter aims to ignite your passion for cancer epidemiology and equip you with the knowledge and resources to pursue a meaningful career in this field. By promoting student engagement and highlighting the vast array of career opportunities, we hope to inspire the next generation of epidemiologists to contribute to the global fight against cancer. Remember, your dedication and expertise have the power to make a real difference in improving cancer outcomes and saving lives.

Conclusion: Advancing Student Knowledge in Cancer Epidemiology: A Call to Action

Congratulations, dear students, on completing this journey of exploring the vast field of cancer epidemiology! Throughout this book, we have delved into the intricate details of studying the patterns, causes, and control of cancer in populations. We hope that this journey has not only deepened your understanding of this crucial field but also inspired you to take action in advancing knowledge and making a difference in the fight against cancer.

Cancer epidemiology is a dynamic and evolving discipline that requires continuous learning and engagement. As students, you are the future of epidemiology, and it is through your enthusiasm and dedication that we can drive progress and make significant strides in cancer prevention and control. This concluding chapter serves as a call to action, urging you to take what you have learned and apply it in meaningful ways.

Firstly, it is essential to recognize the power of collaboration and interdisciplinary approaches. Cancer is a complex disease influenced by various factors, including genetics, lifestyle, environment, and socio-economic determinants. By collaborating with experts from diverse fields such as genetics, biostatistics, public health, and social sciences, you can gain a holistic understanding of cancer and contribute to innovative research and interventions.

Secondly, embrace the potential of emerging technologies and data in cancer epidemiology. The digital age has revolutionized the way we collect, analyze, and interpret data. Stay updated with the latest advancements in data science, bioinformatics, and machine learning, as they offer exciting opportunities to uncover new insights and develop personalized approaches to cancer prevention and treatment.

Furthermore, remember the importance of community engagement and education. As future epidemiologists, you will play a crucial role in disseminating knowledge and raising awareness about cancer prevention strategies among the general public. Empower individuals with the tools and information they need to make informed decisions about their health and reduce their cancer risk.

Finally, never stop learning and pursuing professional development. Attend conferences, workshops, and seminars to stay updated with the latest research and network with fellow experts in the field. Seek mentorship from experienced epidemiologists who can guide and support you in your career journey.

In conclusion, dear students, the field of cancer epidemiology holds immense potential for making a lasting impact on public health. By taking action, embracing collaboration, utilizing emerging technologies, engaging communities, and pursuing continuous learning, you can contribute to the advancement of knowledge and play a vital role in reducing the global burden of cancer. The future is in your hands; let us work together to create a world free from the fear of cancer.

As students in the field of epidemiology, you have embarked on a journey to understand and combat one of the greatest challenges to global health: cancer. Throughout this book, "Advancing Student Knowledge in Cancer Epidemiology: New Insights and Perspectives," we have explored the intricate world of cancer epidemiology, gaining new insights and perspectives that will shape the future of cancer research and prevention.

Cancer continues to be a significant public health burden worldwide, with millions of lives affected each year. As the next generation of epidemiologists, you have a vital role to play in advancing our understanding of this complex disease and developing innovative strategies for its prevention and control.

Through this book, we have delved into various aspects of cancer epidemiology, including the etiology, risk factors, screening, and treatment options available for different types of cancer. We have explored the latest research findings and discussed the challenges and opportunities that lie ahead in this dynamic field.

Our collective knowledge and expertise in cancer epidemiology have grown immensely over the years, but there is still much work to be done. We must continue to push the boundaries of our understanding, embrace new technologies and methodologies, and collaborate across disciplines to unravel the mysteries of cancer.

As students, you have the unique advantage of fresh perspectives and innovative thinking. Your energy and passion can contribute to groundbreaking research and novel approaches to cancer prevention and control. This book has equipped you with the necessary knowledge and tools to make a difference in the fight against cancer.

However, knowledge alone is not enough; action is required. The call to action is upon you, the future leaders in epidemiology. It is time to translate your knowledge into tangible outcomes that will make a positive impact on individuals, communities, and societies.

Engage with the broader cancer research community, participate in conferences and seminars, and collaborate with experts in the field. Seek opportunities to apply your knowledge through internships and research projects. Advocate for policies that promote cancer prevention and early detection. Educate others about the importance of cancer epidemiology and the role they can play in reducing the burden of this disease.

Remember, the fight against cancer requires a multidisciplinary approach and a collective effort. By advancing your knowledge in cancer epidemiology and taking action, you can contribute to a world where cancer is no longer a devastating diagnosis but a preventable and manageable condition.

Together, let us answer the call to action and create a future free from the burden of cancer.